Generis
PUBLISHING

PHYSICIANS' INTERACTION WITH PHARMACEUTICAL SALES REPRESENTATIVES: ETHICAL GUIDELINES

SARDAR MD HUMAYUN KABIR

Title: **PHYSICIANS' INTERACTION WITH PHARMACEUTICAL SALES REPRESENTATIVES: ETHICAL GUIDELINES**

ISBN: 979-8-89248-887-7

Author: SARDAR MD HUMAYUN KABIR

Cover image: https://pixabay.com/

Publisher: Generis Publishing
Online orders: www.generis-publishing,com
Contact email: info@generis-publishing.com

PHYSICIANS' INTERACTION WITH PHARMACEUTICAL SALES REPRESENTATIVES: ETHICAL GUIDELINES

Dr. Sardar Md Humayun Kabir

Contents

Preface

The main objective of this research is to explore the influence of direct-to-physician promotion and moral judgment on physicians' prescription behavior. There are very few studies that have examined to what extent physicians' prescription behavior is influenced by pharmaceutical promotional activities and moral beliefs. This research integrates theories from consumer behavior and ethics to study physicians' prescription behavior in response to pharmaceutical advertising, sales promotion, personal selling, public relations, direct marketing, and moral judgment. The aggressive promotional activities put the physicians in an ethical dilemma and triggered the need for moral reasoning for physicians even when regulatory bodies exist. Hence, this research also studied the role of moral judgment on physicians' prescription behavior and to what extent it moderates the relationship between the behavior and the promotions. The outcome from this research has contributed to new theoretical and practical insights. A primitive contribution has been made by this research at the end of this book by introducing specific guidelines to pharmaceutical marketers and regulatory policy makers for ethical pharmaceutical marketing practices. Finally, it recommends guidelines to physicians' interaction with pharmaceutical sales representatives for establishing ethical medical practices.

CHAPTER 1

INTRODUCTION

1.1. Background

One of the world's biggest and fastest-growing sectors is healthcare. It consists of two industries: the pharmaceutical industry, which produces and sells drugs, and the regulated healthcare provider industry, which offers healthcare services. The pharmaceutical industry, which includes both public and private companies that produce and sell drugs, is a major component of the global healthcare system. Pharmaceutical firms work in both global and local markets, so they must comply with laws, regulations, and policies governing medication production, registration, processing, quality control, marketing, and sales (Pezzola and Sweet, 2016; Alves, Lexchin and Mintzes, 2019; Bazaza, 2020).

The pharmaceutical marketing system in most countries is extremely complicated, involving many governments, advisors, associations, and third-party firms (Goncharuk and Getman, 2014). Physicians, customers, and pharmacists are the primary external partners for pharmaceutical firms in terms of advertisement. Since marketing strategies aimed at patients and pharmacists are minimal, pharmaceutical firms usually target their marketing efforts on doctors (Manchanda and Honka, 2005; Salmasi, Ming and Khan, 2016; Bhatt, 2018; Ahmed et al., 2020). Globally, pharmaceutical companies spent over USD 120 billion in 2016 on drug promotion (Lexchin, 2018; Alves, Lexchin and Mintzes, 2019).

Customers and individuals who use pharmaceuticals are divided into two groups in the pharmaceutical industry (James et al., 2009). Patients are the users, while physicians are the clients. Pharmaceutical companies, in comparison to most industries, are unique and their marketing is heavily reliant on exchanging knowledge to medical professionals under strict guidelines for administering medicines (Shamim-ul-Haq et al., 2014; Murshid and Mohaidin, 2017). Furthermore, administering medicines are classified into prescription and non-prescription types (Ladeira et al., 2011). Non-prescription drugs, also known as over-the-counter (OTC) medications, are marketed to customers without a doctor's prescription and are sold directly from pharmacies (Bazaza, 2020). Pharmaceutical firms rely on prescription drugs for the bulk of their income, and pharmaceutical sales representatives (PSRs) are usually employed to market their drugs to doctors (Brax et al., 2017).

PSRs are the field-force of pharmaceutical organizations. PSRs visit doctors in public and private hospitals, clinics, healthcare facilities, private chambers or medical institutions where health care services are usually given by the doctors to the patients. While visiting doctors, PSRs offer promotional gift items as sales promotion (Rockoff, 2012; Murshid and Mohaidin, 2017). Visiting physicians are also given drug samples and invited to enroll in continuing medical education services by PSRs (Manchanda and Honka, 2005; Rockoff, 2012; Murshid and Mohaidin, 2017). Academics, professionals, and the public are constantly scrutinizing PSR-healthcare professional relationships, which are defended by medical regulatory acts (Fickweiler, Fickweiler and Urbach, 2017; Alves, Lexchin and Mintzes, 2019).

Due to the effect of market share, innovation, and competition from generic drugs, the pharmaceutical industry is rapidly changing (Wozniak, Hassan and Benner, 2012). Pharmaceutical firms make their profit from manufacturing generic drugs. Scientific discovery and development of drugs that prevent or cure diseases and illnesses is the cornerstone of the pharmaceutical industry (Campbell et al., 2007). The pharmaceutical industry's global leaders are the United States, the United Kingdom, Switzerland, and France, which account for half of all sales globally and are known as "Big Pharma" (Anderson, 2014). These international pharmaceutical firms, which mostly supply generic drugs, have distribution offices in the majority of countries.

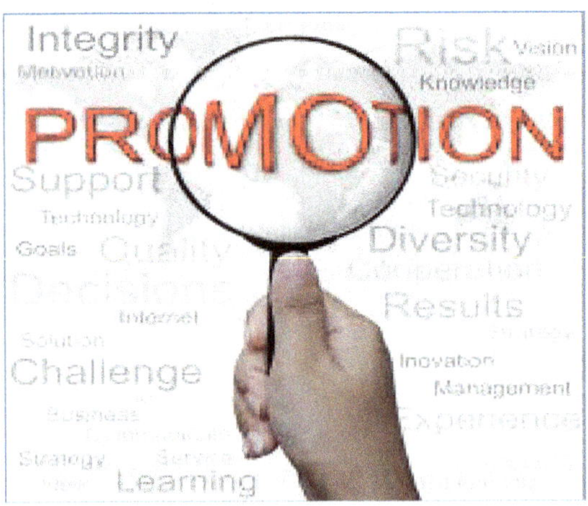

There are many dimensions inside a pharmaceutical promotion directed towards physicians

For instance, here we now talk about the Malaysian context of pharmaceutical industry settings. According to the Malaysian Investment Development Authority (MIDA), there are many multinational companies operating in Malaysia (MIDA Annual Report, 2018). Referring to the Drug Control Authority (DCA) of the Ministry of Health (MOH), the pharmaceutical companies in Malaysia are engaged in the manufacturing of generic drugs, traditional medicines and herbal supplements as well as contract production for MNCs (MIDA Annual Report, 2018). These MNCs are mainly licensed importers such as Pfizer, GSK, Novartis, Sanofi, Eli Lilly, Astra Zeneca. Their medicines are mostly branded drugs and are marketed and distributed by locally incorporated Sdn Bhd (Private Limited) companies. They hire specialized analysts and spend a lot of money on research and development (Jambulingam, Sharma and Ghani, 2009). Clinical trials are typically completed as part of research and development and are overseen by healthcare professionals.

To introduce a new medicine in the market, it requires significant amount of time as permissions are needed in each progression of the production process of medicines. Thus, after many screening procedures and venture during a significant amount of time, pharmaceutical companies launch new products in the market and promote it. They usually target early return on their investment and make associations with the medical doctors for recommending their medications (Latten et al., 2018). There are different levels of doctors based on qualification, reputation, and experience, number of patients and so on which are being characterized by the pharmaceutical companies to recognise their focused clients (Jambulingam, Sharma and Ghani, 2009). In 2012, the pharmaceutical industry spent USD 15 billion on pharmaceutical ads aimed at medical practitioners, according to Cegedim Strategic Data (2013). According to Wei and Delbaere (2015), prescription advertisement interchanges such as free meals and low-value gifts impact physicians' decisions on which drugs to administer. PSRs' advertising practices are covered under medical regulations (Wazana, 2000; Hailu et al., 2021). Pharmaceutical firms also pay doctors in the United States to recommend their products (Guo, Sriram and Manchanda, 2017). This poses a conflict of interest, which is often resolved by governmental policymakers by enacting payment notification regulations. The Physician Payments Sunshine Act (Carey, Lieber and Miller, 2015) created the Massachusetts Open Payment rule, which took effect in July 2009. Data on total expenditure of promotion by pharmaceutical companies are not openly accessible in many nations. That is why most of the published researches on promotional expenditure are US-based because of their freedom of information laws.

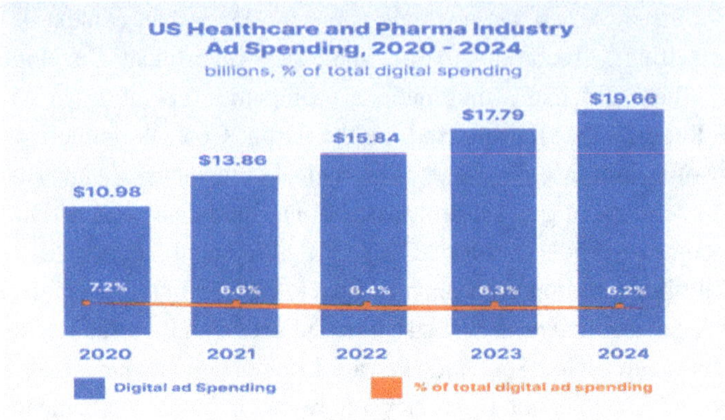

The percentage of total digital advertising spending (in billions) US Healthcare and Pharma industry (Source: eMarketer, July 12, 2022)

The prescribing of drugs is the responsibility of medical physicians (De Lorme et al., 2010). When a doctor prescribes a specific medicine, he is not only suggesting a treatment that can help with a specific disease or ailment, but also deciding about which substance to use (Diehl et al., 2008; Planchon et al., 2009; Kim and King, 2009). The advertising campaigns of pharmaceutical firms have an effect on physicians' prescribing actions. Pharmaceutical firms also create a variety of therapeutic drugs to cure a variety of medical disorders. The standard of treatment determines whether it has a positive or negative impact on the human body. The World Health Organization (WHO) maintains track of drug safety, side effects, trademarks, and prices on a global scale (Pezzola and Sweet, 2016). The International Conference on Harmonization, held in Lisbon, Portugal, recognized and specified consistency, demonstrating the appropriateness of choosing a drug substance or drug product for its intended use in accordance with international drug quality guidelines (ICH, 2015).

In the United States, FDA labs typically test medicines according to the US Pharmacopeia's guidelines. The United States Pharmacopeia (USP) is a research organization that establishes global guidelines for the identification, strength, consistency, and purity of drugs formulated, marketed, and consumed around the world. As a result, pharmaceutical firms put a focus on patient protection of multiple infectious diseases. Nonetheless, pharmaceutical marketers' efficacy in selling to physicians is normally measured by a thorough knowledge of the different variables that affect a physician's prescribing behavior (Hailu et al., 2021; Albarq and Suleiman, 2021).

Pharmaceutical firms have a strong propensity to engage in deceptive advertising campaigns, such as offering discounts and other perks to clinicians for recommending certain brands of drugs (Khan et al., 2016). Profits increase as the number of prescriptions increases. As a result, the physician's ethical or unethical actions as medication deciders are the most important. The two most important performance consequences between healthcare providers and pharmaceutical firms are prescription activity and ethical challenge (Latten et al., 2018). As a result, the primary emphasis of this research is on doctors who write medications and how diverse influences such as pharmaceutical promotion and ethical values affect their decision-making when administering medicines.

1.2. Pharmaceutical Industry in Malaysia

Globally, the pharmaceutical industry is very unique. The foreign generic manufacturers usually let the Malaysian local generic market to become un-ambitious by discouraging the entry of new local generic manufacturers and leaving of small and less-competitive manufacturers (Hassali et al., 2009; MyCC, 2017). Moreover, the Malaysian government only monitors the price of medicine distributed to use in public health sector and allowed the pharmaceutical marketers to decide the prices of medicine for private health sector (Hassali et al., 2009). Under the oversight of the Ministry of Health, the local Drug Control Authority (DCA) is the medical regulatory agency that oversees drug administration (PhAMA Code of Conduct, 2019). In 2014 and 2015, global prescription product sales totaled more than one thousand billion dollars (Statista report, 2015). At the same time, Malaysia's total pharmaceutical product disposal in 2014 was RM 4.7 billion (MOH, 2017). Malaysian pharmaceutical firms manufacture generic medications for Malaysians, and they are mainly listed as specialty drugs, with a sale of around 4.39 billion MYR in 2012 (Piong and Loong, 2014). In Malaysia, there are 75 licensed pharmaceutical companies that produce drugs (Piong and Loong, 2014), and they offer a diverse variety of products in various therapeutic fields. These medicines, manufactured by various firms, cannot always be of similar consistency.

The trends of prescribing medicines in public and private medical centers are different in Malaysia (Kumar et al., 2015). In public medical centers, prescribers usually select generic medicines. But in private medical centers, the majority of physicians had negative perceptions about the safety, efficacy and quality of generic medicines (Kumar et al., 2015). And therefore, physicians in private medical centers usually prescribe with branded medicines (Kumar et al., 2015). While the subject of branded medicines comes, the penetration from manufacturers of branded medicines arises. Like many other countries in the world, the growth of the Malaysian pharmaceutical industry has always been tampered by the strong lobby from branded pharmaceutical manufacturers against generic pharmaceuticals, giving the perception that generic pharmaceuticals are more inferior compared to branded pharmaceuticals (Hassali et al., 2009). For such perceptions, branded pharmaceuticals still dominate the Malaysian pharmaceutical market. Therefore, the branded pharmaceutical manufacturer's product promotions towards the medical doctors in private medical centers in Malaysia need to be studied to see to what extent the promotion influences the medical doctor's prescribing decisions. Also, there is scope for studying the morality of medical doctors while prescribing medicines under aggressive pharmaceutical promotion.

1.3. Medical Regulatory Acts in Malaysia

The Ministry of Health in Malaysia controls medical Acts and Policies. There are many Acts which are initiated, updated and provisioned (Rosnah and Abdullah, 2002). These acts are applicable to West Malaysia, where this research study has been conducted. Some of these Acts are discussed here to understand the research interest better. There are different levels of abbreviation used in legal and ethical records that are only intended for the particular case. It also concerned the individuals, experts, and organizations that were involved in and researched for the purpose of this research.

The Medical Act 1971 explains how the Malaysian Medical Council was formed, led by the Director-General, and how medical practitioners are given permissions to practice. Medical practitioners in Malaysia are required to register themselves with the approval from Director-General. For registration as a medical practitioner, unique requirements are essential. This act also contains requirements demanding medical practitioners to receive a temporary or annual practice license. The Director-General has designated a medical doctor as a Government Medical Officer. Medical students are only permitted to diagnose and treat patients under the supervision of a professionally qualified medical practitioner. The Code of Medical Ethics 2001 covers proper medical practice by doctors to their patients, doctors' professional obligations to their patients, relationships between doctors and other business partners, indirect means of advertisement, and the establishment of a medical practice.

The Medicines (Advertisement and Sale) Act 1956 concerns the banning of advertising related to such illnesses, contraception, ability, or operation. Medicine advertisements must be licensed. Medicine composition must be disclosed. According to the Private Healthcare Facilities and Services Act 1998, any premises where one or more members of the public receive healthcare services is known as a healthcare facility. Health doctors, dentists, pharmacists, clinical psychologists, nurses, midwives, medical assistants, physiotherapists, occupational therapists, and other related healthcare professionals, as well as everyone else engaged in delivering medical, educational, dental, pharmacy, or other healthcare facilities within the Ministry of Health's authority, are called healthcare professionals. Medical, dental, nursing, midwifery, allied wellness, pharmacy, and ambulance services, as well as any other support rendered by a healthcare provider, are examples of healthcare services. This act governs the application for a license to operate or offer health care facilities, as well as the duties of a licensee, holder of the certificate of registration, and person in charge.

1.4. Challenges and Issues in Medical Prescribing

Pharmaceutical firms offer gifts, free dinners, transportation, host conferences, and other incentives to physicians through direct-to-physician marketing, many of which have been questioned as indicators for a physician to recommend medicines (Khazzaka, 2019; Skandrani and Sghaier, 2016). Previous research has shown that pharmaceutical marketing has an effect on physician prescribing behavior, with the majority of physicians accepting gifts from pharmaceutical sales representatives (Zahrani, 2014; Sisugoswami et al., 2018).83 percent of promotion budgets are allocated to doctors (Datta and Dave, 2013). The percentage of spending on promotion was much higher than that on R&D, where promotion was described as the amount spent by pharmaceutical firms on detailing and journal ads (Lexchin, 2018). As pharmaceutical advertisers boost their advertising spending, the price of prescription drugs rises as well (Ibrahim and Bélanger, 2015). According to Business Monitor International (BMI), the pharmaceutical market of Malaysia was worth 6.06 billion MYR in 2012 among which the market share for prescription medicines alone was 4.39 billion MYR (Piong and Loong, 2014). As a result of pharmaceutical firms' ambitious pricing campaign targeted at doctors, overall healthcare spending is growing (Haque, 2020).

The healthcare industry is undergoing dramatic transition around the world. Medical research has seen scientific advances, and the amount of data relating to healthcare systems is rising. The patient's personal records, medical procedures obtained, laboratory results, side-effects, and confidential concerns are all included in this information. Medication complications caused by healthcare providers' cognitive biases are the most serious of these problems (Wittich et al., 2014). It's getting bigger all the time. In developing nations, a substantial number of people have been reprimanded for their medical care. The number of patient reports has almost doubled (Archer and McAvoy, 2011; Bere et al., 2014). Adverse drug reactions are wreaking havoc on the health-care system (Akçura and Zdemir, 2014). These challenges in the healthcare system are eroding people's confidence in doctors (Wittich et al., 2014; Mahmoud, 2016). As a result, patients are moving from one sector to the next (Helble, 2011). In Malaysia, the market for high-quality healthcare is growing, as is customer awareness (MIDA Annual Report, 2018). The partnership between pharmaceutical firms and doctors is at the center of both of these problems.

The role of the physician is vital in assessing whether a patient requires a branded drug or an essential generic medication (Sanyal, Datta and Banerjee, 2017). Physicians also prescribe a nonexclusive remedy. It is usually dependent on branded drugs that use common complex raw materials and function in the body in the same way for patients. It provides the same opportunities and pitfalls as their brand-name rivals (Danchev and Nikolova, 2007). Essential general replacement, on the other hand, will not always be suitable in particular situations where only a branded drug is appropriate for the patient (Bakthavathsalam, 2006). In the other side, if doctors recommend drugs with brand names, prejudices arise (Waheed, Jaleel and Laeequddin, 2011). There is a limited use of generic medicines in the private medical centers in Malaysia which increases the drug expenditure by patients seeking healthcare service in private medical centers and also it reduces the medicine affordability (Kumar et al., 2015).

In developed nations, where the effectiveness of drugs can vary dramatically, the solution of treatments in this way includes several points and can be influenced by various societal views, such as the medication's characteristics and effects (Kim and King, 2009; Joseph et al., 2008). Doctors believe that all prescriptions are of equal quality; as a result, doctors who are heavily influenced by promotions can be tempted to prescribe inappropriate drugs (Waheed, Jaleel and Laeequddin, 2011). Thus, prescription advertising has a direct impact on doctors' prescribing patterns (Zaki, 2014). Pharmaceutical sales executives participate in deceptive business tactics such as bribing physicians in order to reach sales goals (Hirschler, 2013). According to Rahman et al. (2014), corrupt practices have caused a decrease in morals between buyers and sellers. As a result of this interaction between pharmaceutical firms and doctors, the rivalry between a physician's ethical interest and his or her financial self-interest has been scrutinized (Mohiuddin et al., 2015; Latten et al., 2018).

In conclusion, this research is based on the following topic: Physicians play a vital role in deciding which drugs to be given to patients in the pharmaceutical industry. So, pharmaceutical firms spend a significant amount of money on marketing, especially for activities that specifically target physicians, such as supplying gifts, drug tests, conference support, travel expenses, and so on. As a result of these intense campaigns, physicians who are heavily affected by direct-to-physician promotions (DTPP) may be vulnerable to prescribing medications that are less successful, more costly, or not truly required by the patients. It's possible that ethical issues will emerge in this case. Therefore, it's critical to find out to what extent the DTPP influences physician prescribing behavior (PPB) and if moral judgment plays a role in understanding the relationship.

1.5. Significance of Research

The development of theories and models are significant because it offers ideal solutions to specific problems and guides other researchers in conducting further research. Developing theoretical models in physicians' prescription behaviour will bring inclusiveness to the research priorities in pharmaceutical industry (Murshid and Mohaidin, 2017). There are various theories from social and behavioral science that help to understand prescription behaviour (Ahmed et al., 2020). Hence, it is essential to study prescription behaviour to develop an innovative research model.

As like other industries, the driving force for pharmaceutical industry is marketing. Physicians' prescription behaviour is the actual thought of pharmaceutical companies while they market a product (Wazana, 2000). Therefore, pharmaceutical marketers always search for optimal solutions to deal with physicians. Prescription behaviour of physicians depends on various promotional stimuli from pharmaceutical companies. Thus, it becomes significant to study the physicians' prescription behaviour where a variety of promotional factors are being targeted and it is essential to understand the factors that improve physicians' prescription behaviour.

Furthermore, prescription behaviour is a complex phenomenon where the pattern of physicians' prescribing activity is common in many countries with different contextual reasons unique to the region (Waheed et al., 2011; Rasekh et al., 2012).

Hence, there is a need for continuous marketing research in prescription behaviour studies to make valuable contributions to the literature.

This study would aid pharmaceutical company executives in learning more about the common critiques leveled at pharmaceutical marketers and identifying the most effective advertising methods for influencing medical doctors. It would assist administrators in making better use of their advertising budget, lowering promotional expenses and, as a result, lowering the price of the drug.

This research also focuses on medical doctors in order to learn more about their views and where they stand on morally challenging circumstances they faced, as well as what steps they would take in response. It will aid in the development of sound medical practices among physicians, benefiting patients. The detection of ethical issues, as well as their determinants and moderators, will provide physicians with useful information about potential ethical dilemmas. In addition, identifying these unethical behaviors may be useful not just for improving healthcare but also for establishing long-term partnerships with patients (Thomas and Valli, 2006).

Health and regulatory policymakers will be able to monitor unethical activities by physicians and pharmaceutical companies by proposing innovative tactics and pressuring others to agree to them. Understanding the uniqueness of the pharmaceutical industry is vital to growth, as it encourages a dynamic and iterative mechanism for carefully developing a medical data warehouse, which is seen as a requirement for the future direction of the health sector in many countries. In August 2018, Malaysia's Ministry of Health released a list of pharmacy research priorities, signaling the importance of this report. In that list of priorities, treatment decision making by medical professionals has been highlighted (MOH, 2018).

1.6. Scope for Further Research

The prescribing behavior of physicians is multifaceted, with a general definition that encompasses many aspects (Chimonas, Brennan and Rothman, 2007). The problem of doctors' prescribing behavior is also common in many countries. According to Waheed, Jaleel and Laeequddin (2011), such a phenomenon should be taken seriously and researched at frequent intervals. Several factors affect a physician's prescribing actions, including patient-related factors, product-related factors, payer-related factors, environmental factors, and pharmaceutical marketing tactics (Sharifnia et al., 2018). These considerations are usually related to the intensity of the drug, the patient's background, practitioner characteristics, health services, payment type, and pharmaceutical advertisement (Sharifnia et al., 2018). Previous studies combined many of the considerations when determining prescribing conduct, which needs to be properly classified and conceptualized.

Brand equity, brand age, perceived cost, professional impact, physician attitude, demographic variables, expectations, and need achievement are all factors that influence physicians' prescribing behavior, according to previous research (Sanyal, Datta and Banerjee, 2017). Narendran and Narendranathan (2013) found that maintaining a successful relationship with the doctor, arranging seminars, the pharmacy organization's advertising, the quality of the drug, and brand names all have an effect on prescribing actions. Direct mailers, advertisements in technical journals, and low-value gifts (pads, pens, etc.) are also less viable, according to them. However, there are several observations that challenge these conclusions. It is just the pharmaceutical companies' donations to physicians that contribute to drug prescriptions (Waheed, Jaleel and Laeequddin, 2011). According to Waheed, Jaleel and Laeequddin (2011)'s study, the persona of the pharmaceutical salesperson, the nature of the drug, business advertising, and the power of senior colleagues have little impact on prescribing habits. As a result, many marketing methods that must be classified accordingly will influence the choice of medicines.

The marketing mix 4P (product, price, promotion, and place) was developed by McCarthy (1960) and remains the most commonly used method in the marketing field. Promotions, according to Wilson (2005), are the most recognizable face of an organization when it comes to ads. The explicit combination of advertisement, sales promotion, personal selling, public relations, and direct marketing strategies that an organization uses to influentially correspond customer satisfaction and build buyer relationships is referred to as the overall promotional mix, or marketing communication mix (Kotler et al., 2008). These components of the promotional mix were incorporated into Kotler's (2003) buyer behavior stimulus-response model to forecast consumer behavior, which was used in this research to analyze physician prescribing behavior.

Another field where there is an awareness gap is in doctors' prescribing actions. Given the importance of attitude and behavior, researchers should concentrate their attention on identifying additional associations between marketing elements and prescribing behavior. Acceptable prescribing activity is inextricably related to a physician's ethical judgment (Khazzaka, 2019). As a result, the ethical problem that a practitioner faces as a result of pharmaceutical firms' systematic marketing of drug actions must be investigated. Ethics in medical practice is a subject that has gained a lot of coverage in the medical literature (Pellegrino, 1994), and it describes the boundaries between doctors and their associates (Kara-Junior, 2013). It is the morals that preclude a practitioner from taking advantage of his particular situation in order to jeopardize the welfare of a sick patient. The moral is a functional type of ethics that consists of a collection of norms originating from a physician's consciousness and used to govern prescribing conduct (Kara-Junior, 2013). As a result, a well-functioning social community, such as doctors, must be able to judge the morality of prescribing conduct.

There have been significant studies on patient treatment, physician function, and pharmaceutical marketing, but there have been little studies on physician prescribing actions affected by moral judgment. Previous studies did not look at the moral judgment of the medical professionals as an indicator of prescribing conduct. As a result, it has been agreed to fill this gap. In this research, the moral judgment of physicians (Reynolds and Ceranic, 2007; Kara-Junior, 2013) was combined with pharmaceutical promotional tactics. Moral judgment refers to the values that prevent doctors from making decisions that are more beneficial for them than for their patients (Kara-Junior, 2013). Therefore, the moderating role of moral judgment has been investigated in order to better grasp the relationships between the promotional mix and ethical problem of prescribing conduct.

CHAPTER 2

PHYSICIANS' PRESCRIPTION BEHAVIOUR

2.1. Overview

The term "prescribing" refers to the process of establishing a law or action for someone who is undergoing medical care (Merriam-Webster). Sanyal, Datta, and Banarjee (2017) described it as "prescribing decisions" made by physicians in the care of patients. It is described by Ladeira et al. (2011) as "prescription conduct" that demonstrates a relationship between a doctor and a patient, regulated by the physician's (active) act or intervention on the patient (receptor). Physicians' prescribing behavior has been described as behavior that is focused on decisions based on specific knowledge about pharmaceutical firms, their drugs, and the patient's condition (Waheed, Jaleel and Laeequddin, 2011). Prescription loyalty behaviour has been described as physicians adopting the drugs of particular pharmaceutical companies based on evidence of prior effective therapies (Campo et al., 2005) and writing the same brand in the prescription (Waheed, Jaleel and Laeequddin, 2011). As a result, prescription behavior refers to a physician's critical decision to use a medication to treat a condition. It is the result of a physician's decision-making process, which entails choosing the best medication among a variety of choices.

2.2. Physicians' Roles

Physicians' roles in drug decisions are very important. Patients play the roles of purchasers and customers, while physicians play the roles of employers, influencers, watchmen, and policy makers (Abratt and Lanteigne, 2000). As a result, determining how exactly doctors are affected is critical to a pharmaceutical company's success. The doctor plays an important part in prescription advertisement because without a doctor's solution, no remedy can be provided to the customer by the retailer. The doctor is in charge, and his role in disbursement is somewhat unique in that he does not buy or share prescription products with patients. Furthermore, dispensing doctors are an exception, since they purchase the products from the manufacturers and distribute them to customers from their pharmacies. From various outlets, such as clinical texts, different physicians, detail talks by pharmaceutical sales reps, and clinical preliminary results, the doctor comes to consider a pharmaceutical item to cure a particular illness. In some stages of the simple drug behavioral procedure, when selecting a new medicine, the practitioner continues to rely on specific sources rather than others.

As a result, the symmetry of doctors' prescribing behavior is multi-faceted and encompasses many aspects, one of which is "adoption" (Chew et al., 2000; Chimonas, Brennan and Rothman, 2007). Adoption is described by the American Marketing Association (AMA) as: new product recognition, collecting knowledge, forming favorable attitudes toward the product, evaluating it in some direct or indirect manner, finding fulfillment in the experiment, and adopting the product into a standing use or repurchase pattern (Ahmed, Vveinhardt and Štreimikien, 2018; Chren and Landefeld, 1994). Adoption, according to Cialdini (1993), is a social procedure that results in the creation of social affiliations. It is a process of persuasion used in pharmaceutical product promotion to alter physicians' attitudes, behaviors, awareness, and prescribing habits (Ahmed et al., 2016; Clark et al., 1998). Thus, the knowledge, curiosity, assessment, trial, and acceptance phases in a physician's drug behavioral process for choosing a new medication are all part of the adoption procedure. The dispersion process is just as critical as the acceptance process; it is the process by which innovative technologies and products become standards and are adopted by customers.

A recent study of 22 general and specialty physicians in Finland looked at physicians' attitudes toward pharmaceutical product marketing in the context of bringing a new drug to the market (Matikainen et al., 2017). The researchers discovered that the physician-pharmaceutical industry partnership has a positive impact on new drug adaptation. Collaboration occurs here for personal reasons rather than technical ones. Choosing drugs from a related pharmaceutical company is also a major factor in prescription behavior (Janakiraman et al., 2008). It arises as a result of the doctor's confidence in pharmaceuticals. Bednarik (2006) described how pharmaceutical trust can be established and undermined. He (Bednarik) argued that confidence stems from self-expressive (acknowledgement as an expert) product benefits resulting from consistent communication and customer satisfaction. Furthermore, faith in pharmaceuticals grows over time as a result of continued use and beneficial outcomes. Advertisers' responsibilities are restricted to increasing essential needs before to and after medication delivery, as well as giving doctors with useful drug-use advice. The use of medicine in follow-up care is inextricably linked to the success of the first therapy. It seems that keeping track of changes in doctors' conclusions is more challenging.

2.3. Due Diligence

The actions an organization takes to carefully research and confirm a company before starting a business relationship, whether with a client, a third party, or a vendor, are known as due diligence. Due diligence in general form refers to carefully and methodically examining matters that have an impact on the company or on their activities. Previous research has shown that encounters between pharmaceutical sales representatives (PSRs) and medical practitioners may contribute to a conflict of interest (COI), a detrimental shift in physicians' prescribing activity, or a negative view of professionals (Andaleeb and Tallman, 1996; Thomson et al., 1994).

Janakiraman et al. (2008) studied doctor diligence in drug decision-making and discovered essential aspects of caution in drug decision-making. They represented a doctor's current drug judgment as being profoundly affected by previously recommended drugs, and they labeled this auxiliary dependence on subsequent decisions as the "persistence phenomenon" of prescribing actions. They said that doctors don't constantly change their minds; instead, they are either consistent or unrelenting (Janakiraman et al., 2008). Sales marketing and seminar services, according to Janakiraman et al. (2008), may have long-term effects. Doctors with more experience and others who serve in limited healthcare facilities are more likely to be tireless, whereas doctors who are willing to accept promotional items from prescription sales agents are less likely to be consistent (Janakiraman et al., 2008). That means, when it comes to doctors' responses to the progress of medically administered drugs, non-steady doctors tend to be sensitive to defining and seminar meetings, while relentless doctors appear to be approachable only to seminar gatherings, with off-site programs such as lunch or dinner having little effect on the doctor's judgment.

Leo and Kangis (2000) investigated and explained how physicians make decisions on which medicines to prescribe. According to them, one of the purposes of prescription behavior research is to determine the degree to which behavior is solely dependent on the therapist and therefore totally under the therapist's supervision. Therefore, pharmaceutical marketers in the pharmacy industry are increasingly considering medication trends and focusing on physicians' recommending actions (Janakiraman et al., 2008). Since the doctor's opinion on drug management is being more balanced, the aim of promotional communication should be to inform the expert about the medication, its prevalence, and benefits over the existing treatment line. Only when any of the crucial details presented are supported by valid evidence, then the confirmation and assurance to the doctor need to be given (Janakiraman et al., 2008). After receiving the doctor's acknowledgement and confidence about the drug recommendation, the next step is to encourage the doctor to like and accept the brand that the manufacturers support. To do something about the promotion of physician-recommended medications, pharmaceutical advertisers must first understand the medication propensities of physicians and their prescribing conduct (Janakiraman et al., 2008). Physicians' drug preferences change often and rapidly as competitive stimuli change, forcing advertisers to constantly monitor and observe their behavior.

2.4. Decision Making

The "expectancy-value" paradigm and regularizing variables are often used in prescription behavior analysis to explain doctors' drug decisions (Segal and Hepler, 1982). Segal and Hepler (1982)'s model examines expectations for patient outcomes and the value of those outcomes in clarifying drug decisions. While expectancies were included in the standardizing factors, these expectancies were connected to technical and patient-related factors (Harrell and Bennet, 1974; Epstein et al., 1984). In the prescription behavior model, Denig et al. (1988) accepted the dedication to values and attributes. They created a drug decision model focused on the doctor's behaviors, standards, and personal interactions of marketed drugs. The model was studied in the Netherlands, where it was found that coordination of anticipations and qualities regarding drug outcomes, standardizing components, and individual experiences result in a particular medication decision. The results of their investigation suggested that in some areas of drug recommendation, physicians intentionally consider clear benefits and drawbacks when choosing a medicine, while in other fields, the medication choice is taken with less consideration (Denig et al., 1988).

Different fewer recognizing variables can become increasingly important in the above situation. The expressed effect of patient concern on the prescription choice was found to be unimportant among the factors used in their review (Denig et al., 1988). This allows pharmaceutical firms to form close relationships with doctors rather than patients in order to get them to prescribe their drugs, and it also alerts regulatory policymakers to physicians' ethical medical practices. Several reports have shown that pharmaceutical firms manipulate doctors' prescribing actions as part of advertising campaigns while requiring stringent regulatory standards (Lim et al., 2008).

2.5. Interaction between Physicians and PSRs

Pharmaceutical firms have a strong desire to pay doctors cash incentives for recommending exclusive brands of drugs. Benefits increase as the number of prescriptions increases. Drug regulators have proposed training and educational guidelines for sales reps for decades, with the goal of PSRs acting more as collective problem-solvers rather than sales practitioners.

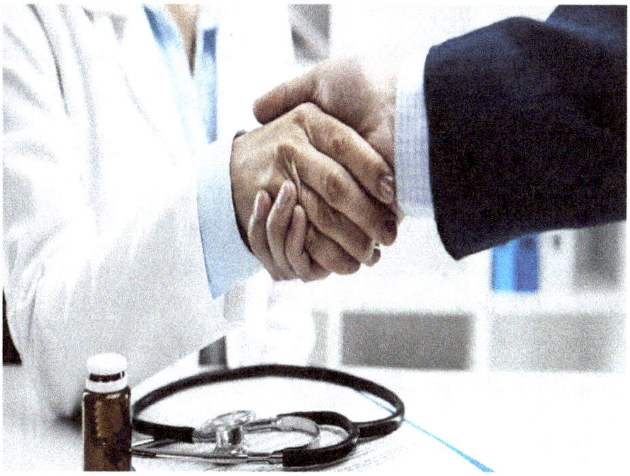

The interaction between a physician and a pharmaceutical sales representative is very common

Caudill et al. (1996) investigated doctors' approaches to obtaining clinical evidence and the ethical influence of pharmacy salespeople in the United States. The majority of doctors accepted that PSRs offered valuable and reliable knowledge on current and historically well-known medicines, but they denied that PSRs played an important teaching part (Caudill et al., 1996). PSRs should not be permitted to work with physicians in places where they operate, according to clinicians (Caudill et al., 1996). McKinney et al. (1990) have investigated physicians' attitudes against prescription promotion and the likelihood of prejudice. Physicians were found to have pessimistic attitudes against pharmaceutical promotion's educational and informative importance, but they did agree on PSRs' impact on conferences and speakers (McKinney et al., 1990). Any doctors are also paid by pharmaceutical firms to offer health care services (Hassali et al., 2009). This is in direct conflict with Pellegrino's (1994) recommendations for joint action on a physician's prescribing conduct. The below are the guidelines:

1. Physicians are first and foremost doctors, not managed-care employees.
2. Physicians must continue to be guardians of patient care quality, and must be considered with any policy, law, or legislation proposed by the managed care agency.
3. Physicians must uphold the physician-patient relationship's dignity as well as a medical practice that is not influenced by societal whims or political decree.
4. Physicians must reject programs that use financial or other benefits to manipulate physician actions in ways that are detrimental to patients.
5. Doctors must constantly prioritize the patient's well-being.
6. Physicians must endorse, support, and engage in clinical effectiveness research.

Physician prescription behavior is a broad phenomenon that is influenced by a variety of influences. According to Shamim-ul-Haq et al.(2014), there are some aspects that affect physicians' prescribing actions. They conducted a study in Pakistan to determine the factors that influence prescribing behavior. They looked at novel drug prescriptions, marketed (generic) products, meeting sponsorships, sales resources, and free drug tests as independent variables. Their results found that when administering a prescription, doctors worry about experimental medicines and are influenced by sales resources and free drug samples. Branded drugs and conference sponsorships had no impact on prescribing habits. Biswas and Ferdousy (2016) discovered that a physician's prescribing behavior is influenced by sales staff involvement, personal relationships, medication efficacy, and business credibility.

In India, Waheed, Jaleel, and Laeequddin (2011) discovered that pharmaceutical firms' market promotion to physicians and the ethical values of medical representatives have a direct effect on physicians' drug loyalty actions. Despite the fact that medical representatives and pharmaceutical sales representatives are also representing the same organization, Waheed, Jaleel, and Laeequddin (2011) distinguished them based on situational factors for controlling physicians. The other factors in that report, such as the consistency of the drug, the pharmacy company's credibility, the likability of physician representatives, and similarity benefits, had little effect on medication loyalty actions (Waheed, Jaleel and Laeequddin, 2011).

Abratt and Lanteigne (2000) investigated the functional relationship between topics relating to prescribing behavior and physician-related influences such as professional impact. The opinion of a physician's senior peers, primary opinion makers, or hospital personnel is referred to as professional influence. Other researchers have argued that senior colleagues play a part in prescribing activity (Bloomfield et al., 2005; Lim et al., 2010; Iyengar et al., 2011). Sanyal, Datta, and Banerjee (2017) investigated the importance of senior colleagues as influencers of the medicine's name, as senior colleagues' effect on prescribing practices varies (Flynn et al., 1994).

According to Williams and Hensel (1991), there has been a substantial decline in the use of PSRs as a source of pharmaceutical knowledge, as well as a rise in the influence of colleagues. Senior peers are expected to be more knowledgeable, self-sufficient, and dedicated members of a local community. By accepting senior colleagues' sessions, the healthcare industry plays an important part in deciding these guidelines (Dumovic and de Vries, 2004). Senior colleagues have the ability to be very important to advertisers in terms of broadcasting the knowledge that pharmaceutical companies want to convey using their products because they characterize faith and value to the customer (Lim et al., 2010), but their professional authority has little effect on physicians' drug loyalty behavior, as Waheed, Jaleel, and Laeequddin (2011) discovered.

Receiving gifts from PSRs raises certain ethical concerns for doctors. Al-Hamdi et al. (2012) conducted a report in Yemen on the impact of pharmaceutical marketing on physician activities and behavior, concluding that all promotional products were sold in return for physicians' prescriptions. Owing to disparities between healthcare facilities and medical procedures, there are restrictions on public and private clinics, staffs, and physicians to judge the price of medications when providing healthcare services to patients and management practices will not be identical in different countries. In a survey comparing Malaysia and Australia, Othman et al. (2015) discovered that the majority of doctors in both countries are likely to change their prescription practices as a result of contacts with pharmaceutical representatives. As a result, the healthcare system is strongly weighted against doctors' prescription actions and is affected by numerous advertising tactics utilized by pharmaceutical firms, putting pharmaceutical sales representatives (PSRs) on the front line. It was concluded that physicians should be better conscious of the effects of their medications (Othman et al., 2015).

A research (Kumar et al., 2014, 2015) on the views of physicians from private medical centers in Malaysia on the use of generic medication when prescribing showed that the majority of the physicians were in favor of generic replacement over brand names, but that generic manufacturers should have more clinical detail. Medicines Australia, Australia's pharmaceutical industry agency, has controlled pharmaceutical firms to ensure that doctors receive continuous medical education (CME), which will improve health care services (Othman et al., 2015). As a result of medication marketing, the physician's decision toward prescribing has a major behavioral effect.

CHAPTER 3

DIRECT-TO-PHYSICIAN PROMOTION

3.1. Overview

In most developing countries, it is now generally agreed that medication marketing must be strictly regulated. Direct-to-physician (DTP) and direct-to-consumer (DTC) pharmaceutical marketing are the two forms. Only the United States and New Zealand accept DTC pharmaceutical marketing beside DTP (Ventola, 2011); the rest of the world allows only DTP pharmaceutical marketing (Manchanda and Honka, 2005). Professional and administrative restrictions are now generally recognized as limiting pharmaceutical firms' sales and marketing practices so that they do not affect patient education, science, policymaking, or prescribing behavior. In this research, physician prescription behavior is described as "prescribing decisions," which refers to medical practitioners' selection of a medication while prescribing for patients in care (Sanyal, Datta and Banarjee, 2017).

3.2. Promotional Tools

Pharmaceutical firms usually intimidate doctors for their marketing campaigns (Manchanda and Honka, 2005; Lim, Kirikoshi and Okano, 2008). Promotional elements, personal selling by pharmacy sales agents (Greene, 2004), free drug samples (Manchanda and Honka, 2005), activities and meetings with doctors, and ads in specialist journals are the most common marketing campaigns aimed at physicians (Bradley and Weber, 2004). Direct-to-physician promotion (DTPP) is described as visits by pharmaceutical sales representatives to physicians, often referred to as detailing (Manchanda and Honka, 2005). Pharmaceutical firms spend the most money on ads to doctors (Wittink, 2002; Hoffman et al., 2009), and detailing has historically been the most effective sales method for pharmaceutical companies (Bradley and Weber, 2004). Despite doctors' claims that detailing is a necessary evil, it clearly has an impact on prescribing behavior (Narendran and Narendranathan, 2013; Khazzaka, 2019). Pharmaceutical firms continue to spend heavily in this form of marketing and have greatly increased their sales force, according to the industry (Manchanda and Honka, 2005).

Pharmaceutical firms engage in advertising campaigns in two ways: they create a pull strategy and a drive strategy (Punchibandara, 2017). The mainstay of the pull policy is mass media promotion, which is banned in many countries. Only the United States and New Zealand allow prescription drugs to be marketed in the newspapers (Buckley, 2006). Many countries where DTPP is more well-known use push as their primary advertising strategy (Wendy and Herman, 2007). The drive strategy, according to Kotler et al. (2008)'s marketing principle, entails "pushing" the commodity across marketing platforms to final customers. It is generally accepted that the average customer is sensitive to marketing communications (Bagwell, 2007). The physician is the "consumer" in the sense of DTPP, and it is their actions that detailing attempts to affect (Dave, 2013). Promotion, according to the convincing view, will influence demand by changing customers' tastes and expectations (Dave, 2013). Furthermore, in the early stages of the medicine's life cycle, there is a lot of confusion about the medicine's efficacy and its characteristics, including the protection study (Narayanan et al., 2005). As a consequence, DTPP is crucial in the early stages of a medicine's launch. Following this early stage, DTPP primarily functions as a persuasion tool, obtaining free samples and reminders from pharmaceutical companies (Chintagunta, Goettler, and Kim, 2012). There are about 81,000 pharmacy sales reps in the United States, and each day they "detail" about 5-10 doctors, demonstrating that the DTPP has a substantial and beneficial effect on physicians' prescribing conduct (Weiss, 2010).

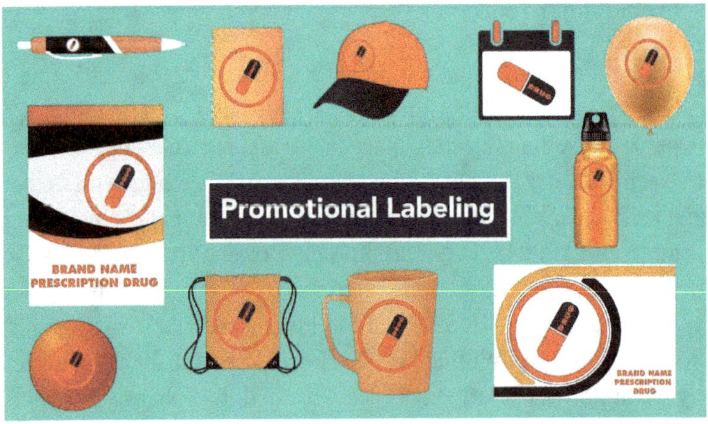

Pharmaceutical marketers promote their medicines by labeling the brand names of their products in everyday use peripherals

Pharmaceutical firms spend more than $20,000 USD per physician per year on outreach activities such as contact calls, incentives, samples, dinners, flights, consulting services, and other expenses (Weiss, 2010). If prescription advertising spending rises and consumer safety concerns become more prevalent, physician-directed marketing campaigns have become increasingly scrutinized by the media. DTPP is considered to have been too harsh and is weakening medical integrity (Lim et al., 2008). The question is also why such marketing campaigns lead doctors to recommend more costly and/or less effective medications when there are less expensive and/or more effective alternatives available. In the other hand, the pharmaceutical industry recognizes that they have useful detail about a medicine's signs, dosage, and side effects, allowing doctors to make smarter decisions (Datta and Dave, 2013). The focus of this discussion is on the consequences of such intervention in terms of how DTPP affects prescribing behavior.

Dey et al. (1999) in India looked at medication marketing and suggested that the object of isolation be linked to pharmacy salespeople and their associations with physicians. They also distinguished other marketing aspects such as advertisement, publicity, distribution, and market analysis. Marketing stimuli (effectiveness of sales force, ads in specialist journals, cost of medication to the consumer, seminar programs) and professional elements (journals, associated experience and teaching, senior colleague's control, recommendations from associates, patient requests) have been described as factors that influence a doctor's prescribing pattern by Abratt and Lanteigne (2000). Mizik and Jacobson (2004) investigated the influence of two main components of pharmaceutical sales practices (specifically, detailing and sampling) on doctors' prescribing behavior and discovered that detailing and free trials had positive and measurably important effects on the quantity of new drugs given by doctors. Ghaith, Aldmour, and Alabbadi (2013) studied prescribing behavior in Jordan, which was heavily influenced by pharmaceutical marketing techniques. It means that pharmaceutical firms are increasingly exposing physicians to a number of competitive stimuli; as a result, pharmaceutical advertisers must consider the factors that affect physician prescription activity on a regular basis. Under such a dynamic climate, keeping on top of marketing campaigns for doctors and knowing the variables that affect their prescription decisions is crucial (Ghaith, Aldmour and Alabbadi, 2013). According to Kotler (1999), marketing promotional strategies were classified under five promotional tools namely, advertising, sales promotion, public relations, personal selling and direct marketing which are being discussed next.

3.2.1. Advertising

Any paying method of non-personal presentation and marketing of ideas, products, or services by an established sponsor is referred to as advertisement (Bennet, 2006). It is characterized as an indirect method of influencing a favorable impression of advertised goods or services by providing information that is intended to influence a favorable impression of the advertised goods or services (Percy and Richard, 2016). Customers' price recognition and evaluation of goods or services improves as a result of advertising (Uusitalo, 2010). As a result, it facilitates brand competition. Instead of merely attempting to reduce the price, the buyer is an aggressive knowledge seeker who behaves rationally by maximizing the total price and search costs (Uusitalo, 2010). Consumer habits and desires are influenced by advertising, which drives demand. Chamberlin's (1933) principle of monopolistic rivalry includes advertisements, demonstrating that ads can help firms distinguish their goods and create an external change in firm-level demand. Advertising increases brand value by communicating advantages and rewards, then reminds and refreshes customers to keep a brand in their minds, resulting in frequent sales and, over time, leading to brand loyalty and franchise (Ambler, 2000). With regard to why consumers can react to ads, three main perspectives (Dave, 2013) have emerged: (1) persuasive, (2) informative, and (3) complementary.

Thus, in the pharmaceutical industry, companies spend a significant amount of money on advertisements to carry out three simple marketing practices, namely, to update, persuade, and inform physicians about the characteristics, benefits, and use of drugs with the goal of positively affecting physicians' behavior (Diehl et al., 2008; De Lorme et al., 2010). When advertising is paired with a superior package of product-quality qualities, it is more efficient (Berndt et al., 1996). Pharmaceutical advertisement plays a different role in the promotion of pharmaceutical drugs since mass-media advertising of pharmaceutical products is banned in most developed countries (Gibson, 2014), leading to major improvements in the strategies used by pharmaceutical firms in product marketing (Al-Dmour, Al-Zu'bi, and Fahmawi, 2013). Advertising strategies will only inform doctors of care choices in this situation. Thus, advertising applies to pharmaceutical firms' marketing of drugs through medical journals, newsletters, and banners at conferences (Ibrahim and Bélanger 2015; Narendran and Narendranathan, 2013). Medicine product literature and brochures are also included in this group (Negash and Adamu, 2017).

3.2.2. Sales Promotion

Sales promotion is characterized as marketing practices aimed at eliciting an immediate response from a target customer by providing value rewards to sales channel participants and/or the final buyer (Belch and Belch, 2007; Ouwersloot and Duncan, 2008). It is often confused with ads because they all aim to raise awareness about a certain promotional deal. The provision of a sort of incentive for a specific action is what distinguishes sales promotion (Arens et al., 2011). It tries to convert optimistic behaviors into behavioral reactions including product trials, repeat transactions, and enhanced product use (O'Guinn et al., 2009). Sales marketing is more time-sensitive and has the potential to manipulate actions (Meo et al., 2014). As a result, the primary goal of sales marketing is to elicit a particular reaction from the target buyer in response to the bid.

Pharmaceutical firms encourage doctors to sell their products by delivering free drug tests and high-value gifts such as rewards for participating in seminars, tourism, CME services, extravagant dinners, honoraria, and low-value gifts such as writing pads and pens (Wazana, 2000; Madhavan et al., 1997; Brett et al., 2003). Sales marketing in the form of high-value presents, such as restoration of a physician's office, sponsorship of a free medicinal camp, sponsorship of patient recognition campaigns, round table discussions, conferences, and symposiums, are all examples of pharmaceutical promotional resources (Shamim-ul-Haq, 2014). Gifts of any kind, whether high or low in value, are more relevant than scientific advertising methods directed at physicians (Boltri et al., 2002). Thus, sales promotion refers to the use of short-term offers to encourage prescription filling (Narendran and Narendranathan, 2013). This domain includes low-value presents such as letter pads, markers, and paperweights, as well as high-value gifts such as laptops, freezers, and televisions, as well as samples of drugs for drug trials (Negash and Adamu, 2017; Ibrahim and Bélanger 2015; Narendran and Narendranathan, 2013).

3.2.3 Personal Selling

Personal selling refers to a special marketing tool where a company's sales team makes a personal pitch to a client in order to close a deal or establish a partnership (Bennet, 2006). It is a part of the promotional mix, and described by Ouwersloot and Duncan (2008) as face-to-face contact in which a sales representative communicates with a customer and satisfies their desires for the shared good of both parties. If a customer is involved in acquiring a product, personal selling brings them to the sales outlet. This process helps the client comprehend the details of the product offering and leads to the product's actual sale. However, not all items are appropriate for personal sale. Personal sales assistants are typically used for complex and costly (industrial) goods (Belch and Belch, 2007). In certain instances, a customer may need additional details before making a purchase and one of the sources the customer will contact is the salesperson. A buyer is frequently drawn to a shopping store after seeing an advertisement in the newspapers. Customers' data demands can't be addressed exclusively by advertising when dealing with complex products or services. The campaign piques the buyer's interest and prompts him or her to contact the firm for more information, resulting in a lead for the sales representative (Ouwersloot and Duncan, 2008).

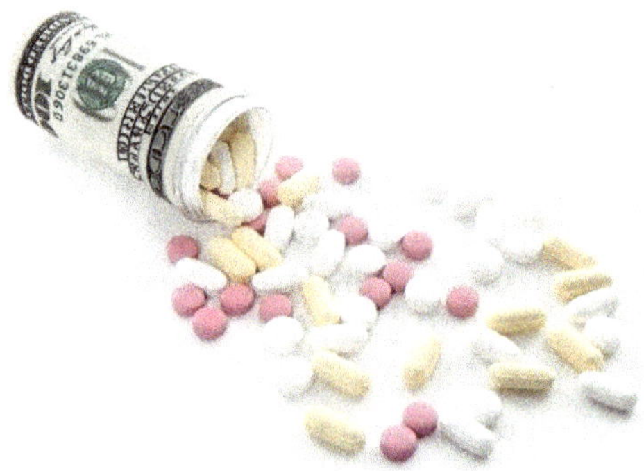

Prescription drugs take unethical exchange for money

Personal sale, according to Brassington and Pettit (2000), is a two-way negotiating mechanism between a company's agent and a person or group, with the intention of shaping, inducing, or reminding them, or sometimes serving them to take appropriate acts. Furthermore, personal sale is crucial in ensuring clients' post-purchase satisfaction and creating profitable long-term purchaser-dealer partnerships focused on confidence and understanding. According to Caris-Verhallen et al. (1997), increased competitiveness within the increasingly changing world of healthcare services has forced pharmaceutical firms to establish and maintain extensive relationships with their clients (physicians). A personal selling session between a sales agent and a physician usually lasts less than three minutes, according to Carter and Chitturi (2009). However, this brief session is extremely successful. Thus, personal selling applies to the amount of information offered by pharmaceutical sales reps as well as the method they employ by visual aids (Narendran and

Narendranathan, 2013). This domain includes PSR relationships, PSR personalities, and PSR visits on a daily basis (Negash and Adamu, 2017).

3.2.4. Public Relations

Public relations is described as developing beneficial relationships with the firm's different communities by favorable exposure, the creation of a positive corporate profile, and the management of negative issues (Bennet, 2006). In general, public relations is a management activity aimed at establishing relationships between the organization and different public groups through contact in order to foster mutual goodwill and a positive image of the company (Arens et al., 2011; Belch and Belch, 2007). Public relations are a vital aspect of announcements to promote intended improvements and development within the organization's internal scopes (Rivero, 2014). It's also used to communicate with external partners in a manner that helps the company's overall communication approach. Good contact is critical in public relations because it has an effect on not just consumers but also other stakeholders. In the promotional mix, public relations play a number of functions (Clow and Baack, 2010):

1. Finding out what people think of organizational reputation, corporate social responsibility, and program execution right now.
2. In partnership with established role players and partners, prepare the approach.
3. Organizing press releases and communicating with the press.
4. Creating official announcements and speeches.
5. Managing media affairs and giving instruction to those who will be making public appearances.

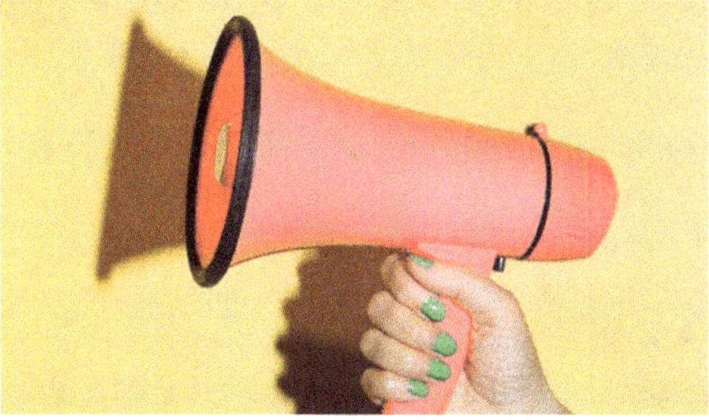

Publicity stunts by top Pharma companies attract more physicians

Several marketing characteristics influence a company's value. According to the Ethisphere Institute in the United States, the amount of a company's worth attributed to real assets has fallen from 90% to just 25% during the last three decades (Brigham and Linssen, 2010). According to other figures, a company's intangible assets (including reputation) today account for 40–60 percent of its market capitalization (Brigham and Linssen, 2010; Gaines-Ross, 2008). As a result, a business's image is one of its most precious properties. People's impressions of an organization are influenced by their prior experiences with it as well as the degree and quality of their contact with it through the media and word of mouth. As a result, it is a combination of various stakeholders' perceptions as well as the realities of its strategies, practices, structures, and results. According to a public relations expert, a person's previous experiences with a brand will account for around two-thirds of their overall impression of the company (Harrison, 2014). Thus, public relations refer to a variety of programs designed to support or defend a pharmaceutical company's brand or individual goods which covers events such as new product launches, conference funding, continuing medical education (CME) programs, and seminar planning (Negash and Adamu, 2017; Narendran and Narendranathan, 2013).

3.2.5. Direct Marketing

Direct marketing entails making direct contact with carefully selected individual consumers in order to receive an immediate response and build a consumer relationship (Bennet, 2006). Direct marketing is a part of the dynamic advertising mix that uses a range of platforms to evoke a response from a network of prospective buyers (Arens et al., 2011; Ouwersloot and Duncan, 2008). Normal postal, phone, radio, printed media, and the Internet are also used in direct marketing. Direct marketing's clever concept allows it to be a coordinated effort of publicizing, advertising, ordering, and distribution. Since the immediate response offering is shown as an advertisement, direct marketing should be considered a form of advertising. According to Ouwersloot and Duncan (2008), coordinated reaction publicizing is a message sent via a mass network that demands an immediate response from a group of people. This structure allows for a higher level of intuitiveness than is possible for traditional mass-media advertising. For example, Internet advertisement includes click-through links that encourage a shopper to tap on an intriguing deal, which will direct him or her to the advertising's website. Typically, the item could then be ordered and paid for over the internet. This also presents the customer with an outstanding preferred place of convenience.

Direct marketing entails responsible and well-received publicity, as it raises visibility and facilitates legitimate transactions. This form of tool facilitates two-way contact so the customer will legitimately respond to the company's message. Furthermore, it allows the organization to determine responses and, as a result, measure the campaign's effectiveness (O'Guinn et al., 2009). Direct marketing has progressed over time, and businesses have discovered cost-effective ways to serve their clients. With the advancement in electronic media and emerging devices, this trend has been accelerated (Subramanian, 2017). Thus, direct marketing refers to delivering product information or advertising directly to physicians via mail, phone, SMS, email, and the internet (Negash and Adamu, 2017; Ibrahim and Bélanger, 2015; Narendran and Narendranathan, 2013).

CHAPTER 4

ETHICAL DILEMMA

4.1. Overview

Several reports have addressed the legal questions around prescribing conduct (Allman, 2003; Sillup and Porth, 2008; Skandrani and Sghaier, 2016). As a result, it is insufficient to forecast physicians' prescription behavior ignoring physicians' ethical dilemmas when administering medicines. The ethical rationale or argument that people use to justify their choices and behavior in morally challenging circumstances is typically the subject of studies that have looked in this chapter at the connection between ethical theory and ethical decision making. These justifications are thought to come from a number of ethical philosophies, each with its own set of basic moral logic requirements (Victor and Cullen, 1988).

4.2. Approaches

The three contrasting approaches to ethical interpretation analyzed by previous scholars were consequential, deontological, and virtue ethics (Baron, Pettit and Slote, 1997; Premeaux, 2004; Lahdesmati, 2005). The intention or goal of an activity is referred to as virtue ethics theory. The morality of an action in regard to its real and future effects was referred to as consequential ethics theory. The intention or goal of the moral assessment, according to deontological ethics theory, is the action itself. Figure 4.1 illustrates how the interpretation of the behavior and its measurement varies based on the analytical methods used.

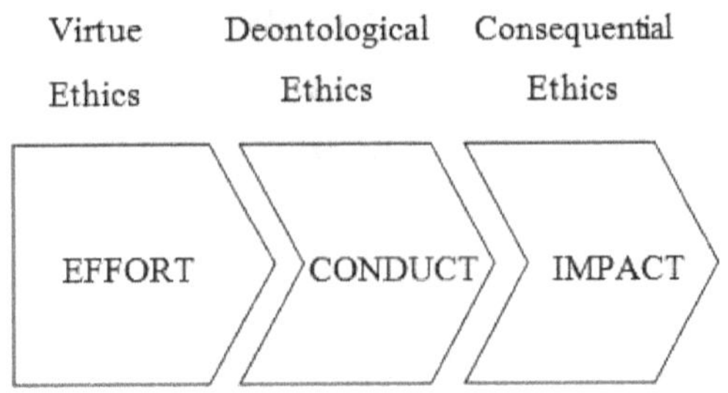

Figure 4.1: Three Universal Approaches of Ethics
Source: (Kaptein and Wempe, 2002)

4.2.1. Virtue Ethics

The object of inquiry in this method is to assess one's own merits, not the act or successes by the consequences that are being judged for the individual in question (Crisp and Slote, 1997). It is concerned with who one is rather than what one can do. A wide variety of attributes can be applied to an individual. These include not only physical characteristics such as age, height, and scale, but also immaterial characteristics such as skills, ambitions, and thought processes (Kaptein and Wempe, 2002). From an ethical standpoint, the second class of qualities is particularly relevant. These traits can be evaluated in terms of how a person can behave in ethically risky situations. It is possible, for example, to describe someone as transparent, truthful, or trustworthy. There are ethically appealing characteristics that are often referred to as spiritual virtues (Kaptein and Wempe, 2002). The aim of this analysis is to evaluate physician behavior rather than to evaluate physicians themselves (person). As a result, virtue ethics is ineffective.

4.2.2. Consequential Ethics

Consequential is a fantastic idea that resonates perfectly with sound judgment (Velasquez, 1992). The results of an action are measured against a particular criterion (the reason or end) in consequential morality. If the effects of an operation are appealing, it is ethically excellent; if they are not, it is immoral. The meaning of this moral theory is that it was formulated specifically to support state policy and legislation, especially criminal law (Kaptein and Wempe, 2002). We continually weigh the consequences for the people participating in our everyday lives. However, there are some flaws in this viewpoint. The need for love, kinship, acknowledgement, health, and a clean environment must be factored into this context to a limited extent - or not at all - in this framework (Kaptein and Wempe, 2002). Where equity can be performed to particular criteria, such as persons' cases to freedom and decency, consequentialists miss the target (Velasquez, 1992). As a consequence, this hypothesis is counterproductive in forecasting physician conduct since the moral content of a physician's acts cannot be predetermined in a global environment.

4.2.3. Deontological Ethics

The expression "deontological" derives from the Greek word Deon, which means "must." Genuine rights must be respected, and uncalled for action must be refused, according to deontological theories, regardless of their consequences (Baron, Pettit and Slote, 1997). Obligation-based or deontological morals address a variety of topics relating to important philosophical hypotheses, such as utilitarianism (Kaptein and Wempe, 2002). Both humans, according to deontology, have some obligations. These duties are irreversible: they cannot be paid off or cancelled. The basis of these obligations is based on different forms of natural rights. Important has no answer to the concepts of rights, obligations, and equity (Kaptein and Wempe, 2002). In either case, this is the point of equilibrium of an obligation-based ethic. According to deontological theory, an action is ethically outstanding if it respects a particular promise (Baron, Pettit and Slote, 1997). Certain persons or groups have rights or a case to equity in such a system. Similarly, a physician's duty (prescribe medicines) requires a range of duties that cannot be ignored. As a result, the deontological ethics principle was used in this research.

Deontology is most closely identified with Immanuel Kant, who argued that the greatest good is good will, and that morally correct acts are those done with a sense of responsibility (Kant, 1998). Individuals use ethical reasoning based on deontology concepts to prevent lying or stealing, according to Reidenbach and Robin (1988); and Granitz and Loewy (2007). Decisions are understood to be focused on structured criteria for behavior in an ethical corporate setting (Victor and Cullen, 1988) and ethical reasoning is required to be based on strict adherence to organizational rules and regulation. The rules of deontology lay out strict criteria for conduct. As a consequence, ethical judgment is thought to be important for moral decision-making and action (Rest, 1986; Pettifor et al., 2000) and it reflects the mechanism involved in the second stage of Rest's (1986) ethical decision-making model, namely judging what is morally correct (Trevino, 1992).

People's moral judgment mechanisms have been discovered in research on moral or ethical reasoning by providing them with abstract moral dilemmas and challenging them to decide what is right or wrong, as well as to justify their decisions. Moral judgment is a strong indicator of moral conduct, as seen in Figure 4.2 (Reynolds and Ceranic, 2007; Guglielmo, 2015; Garrigan, Adlam and Langdon, 2018).

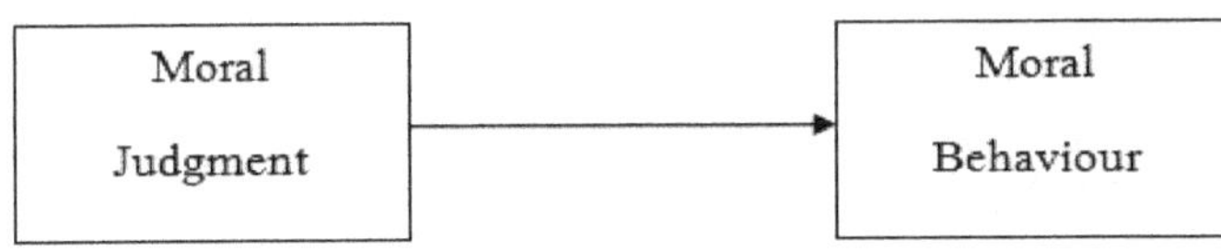

Figure 4.2: Relationship between Moral Judgment and Moral Behaviour

4.3. Moral Judgment

Any action, including judgments, observations, and reaction choices made within the 'judicial sphere,' i.e. decisions about moral issues or values such as right, injury, honesty, and care, is referred to as a moral judgment (Smetana, 2013; Turiel, 1983). An ethical or moral decision can be an answer to an actual or hypothetical ethical question, or it can be a judgment or assessment of the moral tolerability of behavior or the moral existence of others, including person, group, or institutional decisions (Garrigan, Adlam and Langdon, 2018). "Judgments and actions of some kind – including those involving morality – are not a matter of magic, but derive from the interpretation of information," Fiedler and Glöckner (2015, p. 139) wrote. Political judgment, moral logic, moral cognition, and moral decision-making are all concepts that are often used interchangeably (Garrigan, Adlam and Langdon, 2018). Formalism, which falls under deontological or obligation-based approaches to morality, represents moral judgment (Kant, 1994).

The topic of a metaphysical debate is the basis of moral judgment. According to Rest (1986), moral decision-making starts with knowledge of the moral question, followed by a moral judgment, the establishment of an obligation to behave morally, and eventually, moral behavior. Moral behavior is influenced by a number of factors, the most important of which is moral judgment, or judging what is right and what is wrong (Kohlberg, 1981). Ethical predisposition is perhaps the most important option for determining and testing moral judgment (Reynolds and Ceranic, 2007).

The science that asks the question of what is right and wrong in human life is known as ethics (Lille, 1991). Characteristics, actions, and moral standards that regulate person and collective behavior and values are referred to as ethics (Pearsall, 1999). In ordinary market activities, the interaction between consumers and product and service suppliers is crucial. All classes are governed by a code of conduct that must be practiced while doing their duties. Ethics also refers to a collection of beliefs, rules, and moral principles that direct individual actions in social settings, helping people to determine whether or not a human action is right or wrong (Neil and Patrick, 1995).

According to Kant (1998), any action, no matter how insignificant, comes under a particular theory of activity or proverb. There is a proverb for any activity. The crucial difference between behavior and action is the explanation that each activity is ruled by a saying (Kaptein and Wempe, 2002). The object of this circumstance is to decide the correct criterion by which proverbs should or should not be followed. The word "can" implies that this endeavor would be regularized. People will change his beliefs and behavior in this manner at any stage he thinks doing so will result in individual growth or development. It is largely dependent on the circumstances (Kaptein and Wempe, 2002). Several studies have shown that moral judgment has a significant effect on a person's conduct. Moral action is influenced by moral reasoning (e.g., consequentialism, formalism) (Trevino et al., 2006). Moral judgment, according to Rest (1986), starts with knowledge of the moral question. After that, the individual makes a moral decision, declares a desire to behave morally, and ultimately engages in moral actions. The majority of observational research on moral judgment revealed that individuals who consider an action to be exceptionally moral are more likely to partake in the activity (Ajzen and Fishbein, 1980; Hunt and Vitell, 1986). As a consequence, it is possible to propose that moral judgment is inherently related to moral actions in healthcare. Thus, moral judgment refers to a physician's deliberation about different courses of action and choosing of the most morally justifiable (Garrigan et al., 2018).

CHAPTER 5

MODELS AND THEORIES

5.1. Overview

Physician prescribing activity is a dynamic procedure that is affected by a variety of factors. When performing their duties of prescribing medicines, physicians can use a variety of techniques and essential heuristics (Schommer and Hansen, 2005). Theoretical foundations are needed for research on physician prescribing actions. Despite the literature's numerous suggestions on doctors' decision-making, none of the hypotheses can thoroughly justify doctors' prescribing activity and its associated elements (Reyna and Rivers, 2008). As a consequence, numerous hypotheses have been used to see how various factors affect a doctor's decision-making on a daily basis (Buusman et al., 2007). This has culminated in calls for increasingly hypothetical experiments in order to create better mediations that are intended to improve doctors' actions. People are coherent in their decision-making, according to behavioral theory, and so therapeutic methods can be used to explain actions (Ajzen, 1991). A part of recommending that has been tended to by psychological models is a doctor's decision-making technique (Raisch, 1990). According to Godin et al. (2008), further study into the theoretical framework of physicians' prescribing actions is desperately needed. Attitude-behavior theories like Reasoned Action Theory and Planned Behaviour Theory have been widely used in several analyses of prescription behavior (Hemminki, 1975; Gallan, 2004; Raisch, 1990; Godin et al., 2008; Ponnet et al., 2014; Rashidian et al., 2006). The next part follows expand on ideas that prior researchers on drug behavior have used to understand how decisions to prescribe drugs are taken.

5.2. Theory of Reasoned Action

In 1975, Ajzen and Fishbein developed TRA, which is focused on the attitude–intention–action ties and has a high predictive potential of customer behavior (Ajzen and Fishbein, 1975). This is the most well-known model of behavioral motives (Engel, Blackwell and Miniard, 1986). According to TRA, a customer's motives have an effect on his or her conduct. Intentions guide action, where action is the customer's own behavior, which is a function of intention, or his or her eagerness to carry out that behavior. The TRA model, which is linked to the determinants of consciously expected behavior, is well-studied social science model. Reasoned Action acknowledges that certain circumstances (or factors) restrict the impact of attitude on behavior. It distinguishes between behavioral purpose and action by forecasting behavioral intention. It forecasts behavioral intention using two components: attitudes and norms. Other people's beliefs are referred to as norms. As a result, when our behaviors lead us to do one thing, but the relevant norms lead us to do something different, both aspects have an impact on our behaviour. The mood and desire to succeed, according to TRA, motivates social conduct.

The behavioral intentions model of Ajzen and Fishbein (1980) is based on the principle that consumers in a cognizant and conscientious design will first form convictions about the individual properties of an object, and then carefully consolidate these convictions to form a general disposition about the item. In this way, the model's focal point is on the buyers' conscious mindset, based on verbal data as perspective, that is, the buyers' contemplations or convictions about the products, such as buying a particular brand, which has been resolved as one of the courses of attitude growth and improvement, referred to as the focal path, or the systemic planning process (Loudon and Bitta, 2002).

In any case, buyers form attitudes through a variety of procedures that do not depend on a conscious and purposeful concept, such as the fringe course or the heuristic handling scheme, in which buyers shape attitudes by pairing the object being responded to with seemingly unrelated motives (Loudon and Bitta, 2002). The buyer's component of contribution and capacity to process knowledge have affected the option of path, focal or fringe, by the consumer, the individual for attitude growth or change. The model indicates that if the buyer's association levels are high, suggesting a high degree of personal value, the buyer will be able to consider recognize the item and its qualities, and the focal course will most likely be chosen (Loudon and Bitta, 2002). When the degree of correlation is poor, monetary implications are not overly important to the buyer, so elaboration is unlikely, and the buyer would most likely be influenced by factors unrelated to the object in question (Loudon and Bitta, 2002).

Davis (1989) developed TAM (Technology Acceptance Model) based on TRA to describe the use of personality structure at work. TAM used TRA's fundamental relation to explain the influence of external influences on a person's behaviors, internal beliefs, and intentions. TAM takes into account the impact of two factors: perceived advantage and perceived ease on attitudes toward use, and thereby behavioral intentions and real use (Davis, 1989). TAM was used by Sanyal, Datta, and Banerjee (2017) to recognize a few improvements in physician prescribing actions. They (Sanyal, Datta, and Banerjee) demonstrated that for a given treatment, physicians normally select both branded and generic medicines that are equally successful. This model, however, cannot be used in cases where pharmaceutical marketing techniques affect physician prescribing actions.

5.3. Theory of Planned Behaviour

TPB is an extension of the TRA that adds perceived behavioral influence, as well as mood and contextual standard, to give the principle a wider scope. When trying to alter or affect doctors' prescription actions, the TPB is one of the most appropriate and commonly applied behavioral hypotheses (Eccles et al., 2012). The TRA has been shown to have broad acceptance in a number of user corporate environments, with the caveat that it was structured to resolve activity that is solely under an individual's volitional power. To counter this restriction of the TRA, Ajzen (1988, 1991) suggested an expansion in the form of the TPB to address behavior that was not always under voluntary supervision. With the inclusion of the perceived behavioral control (PBC) construct, the TPB is identical to the TRA. The PBC is regarded as explicitly evaluating intentions as well as behavior in the TPB.

PBC refers to a doctor's assessment of how easy or difficult it is to carry out a certain behavior. The influence of causes that can promote or spoil the difference in behavior is attributed to PBC (for example, prescribing). Attitude reflects one's emotions about something, and it may affect one's "inclination or actions" to behave in particular ways. To be more precise, attitude applies to a doctor's favorable or unfavorable attitude toward marketing practices that affect their prescribing. Physicians' attitudes toward prescription firms' lobbying practices will assess their prescribing behaviors. The TBP showed a high capacity to forecast doctor actions in the healthcare environment in a meta-analysis led by Godin et al. (2008). TBP has shown to be a useful systemic theory for dealing with the factors that influence prescribing behavior (Ponnet et al., 2014; Kramer et al., 2014; Perkins et al., 2007). However, Godin et al. (2008) showed that the TPB paradigm has a few shortcomings, namely, the system does not take the emotional response into account (Lee and Yun, 2015). Furthermore, Conner and Armitage (1998) called for the inclusion of cognitive variables as a central component of expanding behavioral hypotheses. TPB was used to explain the dual position of a doctor as a customer and advisor, as well as to get a greater understanding of how doctors respond (Groves, 2006). The TPB is strongly associated with the doctor as a professional in a clinical setting (Godin et al., 2008). Regardless of their position, physicians are still the focus of comprehensive pharmaceutical marketing campaigns and are studied in terms of persuasion theory and stimulus-response theory (Murshid and Mohaidin, 2017).

5.4. Persuasion Theory

In drug behavior research, persuasion theory is used to identify better ways of offering interferences to change physicians' prescribing behavior, such as marketing activities (Raisch, 1990). The principle provides a solid foundation for answering research questions about medicinal marketing in the form of drug prescribing (Schommer and Hansen, 2005). Persuasion necessitates that a person's actions alter eagerly in reaction to a given stimuli, and therefore the mind modifies the interaction (Bettinghaus, 1980). In most cases, this mental shift is linked to a person's unique needs (physicians) and their requirements (e.g., prescriptions needed by their patients). Persuasion has an impact on everyone on a daily basis, whether it's by decision-making authority or a constructive effort to persuade or manipulate (Schommer and Hansen, 2005). Persuasion is often described as "human communication aimed at influencing others' philosophies, values, or points of view" (O'keefe, 2002). Persuasion is a concept that includes both emotional and cognitive reactions to a situation in which individuals find themselves. Persuasion is a mechanism in which intellect and motivation combine to affect an individual's actions against a target. Persuasion has four main dimensions of theory: (1) the sender of information (e.g., pharmaceutical company representatives), (2) the receiver (e.g., a physician), (3) the interactive or active exchange between the sender and receiver, (4) the modification of behavior (e.g., prescription behavior), which may be voluntary, and there is a certain amount of time required for the contract.

In the context of persuasion theory, the Elaboration Likelihood Model (ELM) is the most commonly used model (Petty and Cacioppo, 1986). Elaboration entails participating in important-issue logic (O'keefe, 2002). People can use both subjective capacities and emotional responses to interpret facts and make decisions, according to the model. The ELM model demonstrates that the source of data (salespersons' promotional efforts) and the manner in which it can be offered, as well as the beneficiary characteristics, can affect the understanding of the data needed to make decisions, and thus influence behavior (Petty and Cacioppo, 1986). The ELM model is made up of two types of control strategies: core and periphery. The core strategy implies an irregular state of preparation and mental exertion, while the fringe strategy entails a lower degree. Petty and Cacioppo (1986) proposed that as less participants are involved in a scenario, they pay less attention to the evidence presented and are less likely to argue subjectively (Schommer and Hansen, 2005). Fortunately, when the issue's result is bad, the terminal's approach becomes increasingly important (O'keefe, 2002). As a result, doctors could be influenced in the same way that any highly active user who may integrate data and, as a result, accept broad subjective processing, as depicted by the ELM model (Petty and Cacioppo, 1986).

5.5. Stimulus-Response Theory

Kotler's (1997) buyer behavior stimulus-response (S-R) model is similar to the ELM model in that both require emotion and perception to persuade an individual. This person is the physician in drug behavior tests. This paradigm is related to behaviorism's black box principle. The fundamental relationship between the stimulus and the resulting reaction is important here, not the processes that the consumer goes through (Xing and Othman, 2015). The black box model explains the relationship between inputs, consumer attributes, decision-making, and customer reactions. Marketing stimuli are designed and processed by companies, while environmental stimuli are generated by technological, economic, cultural, and political factors (Kotler, 2004). This new paradigm, which builds on material generated in the behavioral sciences, focuses on the decision process that consumers go through while evaluating goods and services. It focuses on the emotional process that takes place before and after a buy.

The stimulus response model of consumer behavior (Kotler, 1997) is useful for understanding individual consumer purchasing behavior in the form of individual consumers buying consumer goods. Individual consumers are exposed to marketing stimuli such as product, price, place, and promotion, as well as other stimuli such as fiscal, technical, political, and cultural dimensions, according to the model. The buyer's internal processes are represented as a black box, with observations of buyer decisions such as product range, brand selection, dealer selection, purchasing quantity, and timing. The stimulus-response model is depicted in Figure 5.1.

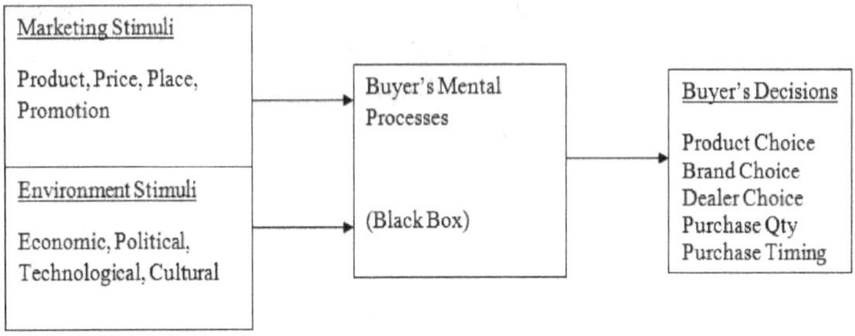

Figure 5.1: The Basic Buyer Behaviour Stimulus-Response Model
Source: (Kotler, 1997)

A practitioner, as a client, is exposed to all of the same influences that a person might experience when making a normal buying decision. According to the S-R model, a stimulus paired with proper adjustment and a particular population would result in a response that the vendor can forecast. Advertisements, product advertising, public relations, personal selling, and direct marketing (Kotler, 1999) are some of the pharmaceutical promotional combination variables that penetrate the "black box" known as the customer (i.e. the physician) and produce some positive responses/purchases. All of these stimuli join the buyer's black box, where they are transformed into a set of observed responses. A pharmaceutical corporation, on the other hand, is interested in learning how inputs are converted into responses inside the consumer's black box, which is divided into two sections (Kotler, 2003). To begin, the buyer (physician) properties can influence how marketing motivators consume, imagine, and perceive stimuli. Second, the buyer's (physician's) decision-making process can eventually decide what, if any, purchasing (prescriptions) activity happens (Figure 5.2).

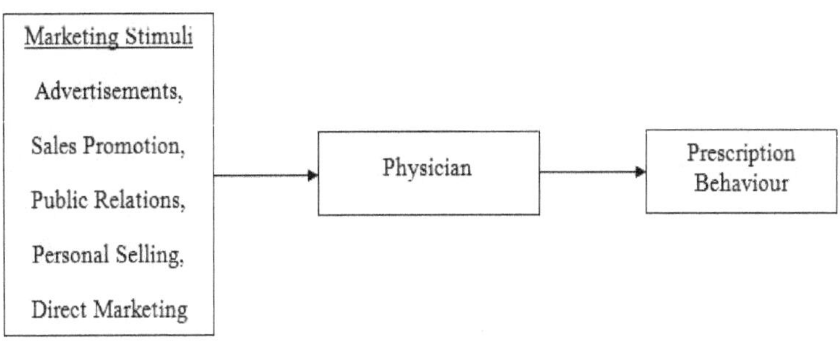

Figure 5.2: Proposed Physicians' Prescription Behaviour Adapted from Buyer Behaviour Stimulus-Response Model of Kotler (2003)

In Figure 5.2, marketing stimuli refers to Direct-to-Physician Promotion (DTPP) which includes Advertising, Sales Promotion, Personal Selling, Public Relations and Direct Marketing. The following chapter will further discuss the relationships among DTTP and its elements with physicians' prescription behaviour.

CHAPTER 6

Interralations and DISCUSSION

6.1. Overview

This chapter provided a complete discussion of the research constructs explained in earlier chapters. The findings were discussed with theoretical background and previous empirical results. The discussion is narrated through a few sections which describes the influence of direct-to-physician promotion (advertising, sales promotion, personal selling, public relations and direct marketing) by pharmaceutical companies towards physician's prescription behaviour. This chapter explicitly elaborates the significance of promotional mix elements directed towards physicians. It also describes the significance of moral judgment on physician's prescription behaviour and describes the moderating role of moral judgment between direct-to-physician promotional elements and physicians' prescription behaviour. The objective of this chapter is to get the answer of the main research question which was "to what extent direct-to-physician promotion (DTPP) influence physician's prescription behaviour (PPB) and does moral judgment (MJ) play any role in understanding the relationship".

6.2. Direct-to-Physician Promotion and PPB

Promotional mix is the planning, preparation, execution and monitoring of integrated communication strategies. Pharmaceutical companies engage different stimuli through promotional mix elements which influence the physician's prescription decision making process (Ahmed et al., 2020; Khazzaka, 2019). According to Kotler (2002), physician features influence the way in which stimuli are perceived, fictional, and interpreted through the promoters. The process of decision making by the physician ultimately defines the physician's prescription behavior (Kotler, 2005). Therefore, in this research based on Kotler's (2002) buyer behaviour: stimulus-response (SR) model, the pharmaceutical company's promotional mix elements has been taken as stimulus factors for getting physician's response. Typically, pharmaceutical company's promotional mix elements are advertising, sales promotion, personal selling, public relations and direct marketing (Murshid and

Mohaidin, 2018; Ahmed et al., 2018, 2020; Alowi and Kani, 2018, 2019). Here, the research was carried out to find the extent to which these promotional mix factors directed towards physicians (DTPP) influence physician's prescription behaviour (PPB). The finding has been mostly compared with other empirical studies conducted in developing countries.

6.2.1. Advertising and Physicians' Prescription Behaviour

According to theory, advertising significantly and positively influences physician's prescription behaviour. This result is in-line with previous study results by Mohammed and Kheder (2019); Ahmed et al. (2018); Negash and Adamu(2017); Biswas and Ferdousy (2016). But it is contradicted with the results obtained by Sharifnia et al. (2018) where the researchers found that pharmaceutical advertising have no effects on physicians' prescription behaviour in Iranian context. It might be because, Sharifnia et al. (2018) investigated advertising directed towards physicians along with advertising directed towards consumers which are not in the scope of this study. Direct-to-Consumer Advertising (DTCA) is allowed limitedly in very few countries. That's why the country context can represent different results for advertising. The information carried out through pharmaceutical advertisements is a major concern by different national health regulators and there are differences in the extent to which national laws are imposed.

Pharmaceutical product advertising insists a dual role by enhancing the knowledge of the physicians and increases awareness. Advertising disseminates the product information which establishes more acceptance level of drugs by the physicians. Medical journals, healthcare magazines, product brochures, leaflets, and banners played a significant role in shaping the prescription behavior of physicians. It is a significant window of opportunity to enhance the awareness of a product and increases the influence on physicians; thus, pharmaceutical advertising has been revealed as a competitive predictor. Pharmaceutical product advertising in reputed medical journals like American journal of medicine, British medical journal, Lancet, JAMA, etc. influence physician's prescription behaviour (Ahmed et al., 2018). Medical journal advertising has been found very competitive for new drugs (Dixon et al., 2011).

6.2.2. Sales Promotion and Physicians' Prescription Behaviour

That means, sales promotion significantly and positively (according to theory) influences physician's prescription behaviour. In pharmaceutical promotional activities, sales promotion includes offering low and high value gifts, free medical equipment, free drug sample and sponsorship to conferences. Low value gifts mean pens, paper weights, writing pads etc. and high value gifts mean laptop, television, freezer etc. Sponsorship to conferences includes local and international events. Sales promotion by pharmaceutical companies and physician's prescription behaviour has a strong relationship. In a study on effects of gifts on physician's prescribing behaviour, the researchers stated that the matter of obligation occurred by offering low value gifts cannot be misjudged as even coffee mugs can have a big effect (Katz et al., 2003). In this study, sales promotion has been identified as the most effective tool in influencing physician's prescription behaviour. Physicians are more likely to be influenced by sales promotion while prescribing any products, because they gain a direct monetary benefit in the form of gifts. So, pharmaceutical companies understand that it is obligatory for physicians to prescribe their products. Therefore, sales promotion is a potential source of responsiveness by physicians.

6.2.3. Personal Selling and Physicians' Prescription Behaviour

Personal selling significantly and positively (according to theory) influences physician's prescription behaviour. According to Kotler (2002), personal selling is an expensive tool among the other communication channels. Pharmaceutical promotional activities through personal selling are carried out by pharmaceutical sales representatives (PSRs). Drug information are detailed to physicians by PSRs during their visit. Detailing is a form of personal selling which impact the relationships between pharmaceutical companies and physicians. While meeting with the physicians, PSRs eventually make the physicians to prescribe his/her company's product based on maintaining regular communications and follow up meetings. Personal selling includes daily visit of PSRs, weekly visit of senior PSRs, personality of PSRs, personal relationship of PSRs with physicians and skillful detailing of PSRs. By visiting physicians regularly, PSRs can make better relations with the physicians which leads to maximum prescription generation. It is a powerful tool of promotion, although physicians usually deny their relationship with PSRs (Workneh et al. 2016). In this study, personal selling has been found to be the least important factor. The definition of personal selling used in this study trailed the descriptions by Kotler

(1999). Personal meetings with physicians are usually carried out by the help of visual aids, literature, laptop or tablet.

6.2.4. Public Relations and Physicians' Prescription Behaviour

Public relations significantly and positively (according to theory) influence physicians' prescription behaviour. Public relations assist a company and its customers to interact with each other. It comprehensively applies to companies as a shared gathering, not only a business; and publics include the wide range of partners. Public relations are utilized for long-term goal of company-image creation, emerging productivity and upholding the company name, to improve overall marketing exercises. It is a strategic component of the promotional mix elements. Previous studies identified that the best effective and important strategy which influence physician's prescription behaviour was public relations of the company (Khajuria and Khajuria, 2013; Gupta et al., 2018; Biswas and Ferdousy, 2016). In this study, public relations is found as the second most important factor which includes activities like new product launching ceremony, continuous medical education program, round table discussion program, invitation to conferences and reputation of the pharmaceutical company.

6.2.5. Direct Marketing and Physicians' Prescription Behaviour

Direct marketing does not influence physician's prescription behaviour which contradicted slightly with previous study results by Mohammed and Kheder (2019); Biswas and Ferdousy (2016) where both the study found it least effective. Direct marketing is the communication between the buyer and the seller to inform the buyer about the product for getting sales as the main objective. Direct marketing pursues action from a specific group of customers considering a correspondence from the advertiser. That's why it is sometimes mentioned as a type of advertising. The correspondence can be made by different methods like telemarketing, direct email marketing, postal mails etc. For pharmaceutical business, buyer is the physician who prescribes medicines resulting sales and seller is the pharmaceutical company itself. Pharmaceutical companies usually send product information to the physicians using post, phone, email or other channels. In this study, direct marketing includes direct phone call, short messaging service (SMS), mobile applications, e-mail and postal mail. But, the relationship between direct marketing and physician's prescription behaviour was not found significant. It might be because physicians do not entertain direct marketing communication from pharmaceutical companies due to their busy schedule. Therefore, direct marketing does not influence physician's prescription behaviour.

6.3. Moral Judgment and PPB

Moral judgment is favorable to good moral reasoning as one must decide for oneself what is good and bad, right and wrong. One must ensure to make the right choices while taking any decisions. Historically, researchers have addressed this issue for personal and professional behaviour. Ethical behavior, particularly in professional lives depends on moral reliability which is, being capable of acting on sound moral judgments (Schaefer and Savulescu, 2017). As there are too many ethical issues surrounding the pharmaceutical promotional activities directed towards physician's decision making (Zetterqvist, Merlo and Mulinari, 2015; Othman et al., 2015; Mohiuddin et al., 2015; Skandrani and Sghaier, 2016; Khan et al., 2016; Khazzaka, 2019; Mohammed and Kheder, 2019), it is very crucial to identify the influence of moral judgment on physician's prescription behaviour. Moral judgment significantly and positively influences (according to theory) physician's prescription behaviour. In prescription behaviour studies, the use of moral judgment is almost new. That's why this research is a primitive for physician's prescription behaviour studies. Selection of moderator depends on theoretical background with literature support (Frazier et al., 2004). Although, moral judgment has rarely been used in prescription behaviour studies, it acts as a moderator in various types of research (Ferrell and Gresham, 1985).

6.4. DTPP, MJ and PPB

The physicians get to know about the pharmaceutical products from different sources like book of medicines, clinical reports, detailing by pharmaceutical sales representatives and so on. The physicians appear to depend on specific sources at specific phases of the dynamic procedure while choosing a specific medication. The physician's choice procedure on the determination of another medication goes through different stages like mindfulness, intrigue, assessment, preliminary and selection. During promotion of pharmaceutical items, the physician's role as a prescriber is vital as the right choice of medicines dispensed to the consumers depends on the prescription. Thus, the physician's indirect role of dispensing medicines largely influence by the moral judgment of this action.

6.4.1. Advertising, MJ and PPB

According to World Health Organization's ethical criteria, specific information of healthcare products should be demonstrated in the pharmaceutical advertisements for healthcare professionals to understand correctly (WHO, 1988). In Bangladesh, 34% of product information in a sample of 116 brochures for family physicians has been found misleading (Islam and Farah, 2007). In Nepal, drug advertising materials provided to physicians in the hospital failed to mention adverse effects which can cause health degradation for patients if prescribed by the physicians (Alam et al., 2009). In Sri Lanka, the scientific research information mentioned in the drug promotional materials were found of poor quality (Kommalage et al., 2016). In India, majority of drug promotional literature collected from physicians in hospitals failed to satisfy the WHO criteria for rational drug promotion (Ganashree et al., 2016). A comparative study among Malaysia, Australia and United States on the pharmaceutical advertisements in medical journals discovered that most of the claims were unclear and of poor quality (Othman et al., 2010). Moreover, pharmaceutical companies spend huge money in different clinical studies to get published in reputed medical journals with their favorable results of a medicine (Chren and Landefeld, 1994; Couturier et al., 2000). Therefore, unethical conduct by pharmaceutical companies triggers the necessity of judgment by the physicians on moral ground.

6.4.2. Sales Promotion, MJ and PPB

Sales promotion is an important ethical concern for physicians. It acts as an incentive for physicians (Skandrani and Sghaier, 2016). The incentives in the form of gifts from high value to low value possess huge obligation for physicians to accept and work on it. Sponsorship to medical congresses and events also comply the same. While pharmaceutical companies spend millions of dollars in providing gifts, they expect more in return. While physicians are accepting such gifts, they fell in an obligation to return the favor by prescribing more products resulting sales. This type of exchange is considered as unethical (Haines and Olver, 2008; Latten et al., 2018). According to Skandrani and Sghaier (2016), some physicians stated that these practices are unethical and unacceptable where others stated as purely commercial or common. According to World Health Organization, promotion of pharmaceuticals has been defined as, "all informational and persuasive activities by manufacturers and distributors, the effect of which is to induce the prescription, supply, purchase and/or use of medicinal drugs" (WHO, 1988). In Malaysia, the promotion of prescription medicines by pharmaceutical companies is self-regulated. The Pharmaceutical Association of Malaysia (PhAMA) code of conduct is intended to comply with the legislations provided by Ministry of Health. This code of conduct provides morals for the ethical promotion of pharmaceutical products to healthcare professionals. There are differences between the regulation mentioned in the industry Codes of Conduct and the actual conduct of the industry (Zetterqvist, Merlo and Mulinari, 2015). Therefore, sales promotion will influence more on physicians' prescription behaviour if physicians apply moral judgment in their action.

6.4.3. Personal Selling, MJ and PPB

Numerous research studies have confirmed the dominance of pharmaceutical sales representatives (PSRs) through personal selling as a promotional tool for marketers in terms of influencing physician's prescription behavior (Matikainen et al., 2017; Othman et al., 2015; Salmasi, Ming and Khan, 2016). There are regulatory guidelines for physicians and PSR's interactions, but general practitioners (GPs) who meet PSRs more often were potentially less likely to follow these guidelines (Brax et al., 2017). Physicians, who maintain positive and active relationship with PSRs, are the early adopters of new drugs with product advantage whereas those who does not maintain such relationship, relies on therapeutic advantage (Matikainen et al., 2017). Although, the pharmaceutical industry is curving the total number of sales representatives, most physicians intended to see PSRs as reported in a study by Mack (2014). About two-third of 446 physicians stated that their prescription behaviour did not affected by PSRs, but half of the physicians reported that they met PSRs every day for fifteen minutes or more (Guldal and Semin, 2000). It has been found that PSRs provide misleading information consistently while giving oral presentations to the physicians in their meeting (Mintzes et al., 2013). Hiding scientific information or efficacies is the reason for gaining market share of the product. But it is obvious that this type of conduct is unethical, and physicians should be avoiding such interactions with PSRs. Therefore, it can be said that PSRs personal selling attributes will influence more on physicians' prescription behaviour if physicians apply moral judgment in their action.

6.4.4. Public Relations, MJ and PPB

The relations between physicians and pharmaceutical companies become stronger through publicity events like continuous medical education programs, round table discussion programs, new-product launching ceremonies, scientific seminars and conferences. The pharmaceutical companies spend money for significant medical breakthroughs and catch the attention of the healthcare community to change the perception of treatment of a disease (Stafford et al., 2004; Hersh et al., 2002). From March 2007, public health department of France has regulated healthcare professionals to declare their financial ties with pharmaceutical companies. Even with that requirement, a physicians' organization along with a consumer group have placed charges against nine key opinion leaders (KOLs) who were well-known in medical field and failed to disclose their links with pharmaceutical companies while speaking in a public event (Lenzer, 2016). Majority (75%) of Australian medical experts stated that they receive invitation regularly to new product launches, symposia or educational events from Pharma companies (McNeill et al., 2006). Such events strongly influence physicians' prescription behaviour. Hence, Medicines Australia always monitors such promotional activities and expenditures to reduce unethical sanctions towards physicians (Medicines Australia, 2007). In a study, 63% of general practitioners in Malaysia said that they received invitation to a company-sponsored program, 70% of general practitioners has been offered continuous medical education programs (Othman et al., 2015). According to De Ferrari et al. (2014), activities perceived to be more ethical were the continuous medical education program (68.9%). The result of the study by De Ferrari et al. (2014) indicates that physicians make distinctions about ethical appropriateness of different types of pharmaceutical programs. Therefore, it can be said that pharmaceutical company's publicity will influence more on physicians' prescription behaviour if physicians apply moral judgment in their action.

6.4.5 Direct Marketing, MJ and PPB

Direct marketing tools such as pharmaceutical product information placements in email, SMS, postal mail, direct phone call and mobile applications influence physician's prescribing habits (Henderson et al., 2008; Prosser et al., 2003). Direct e-mail campaign played a significant role as a direct marketing tool initially. According to Ransom (2017), a pharmaceutical company allocated $851,000 for a direct mail campaign in the US (105 e-mails to each physician for a given time period). Direct mail content usually includes invitation letters, greetings, product brochures, event notifications all are in the form of pharmaceutical product advertising directed towards physicians. A top physician could get two to three mailings every day throughout a calendar year (Ransom, 2017). A study revealed that there were 741,213,700 direct mails were e-mailed and about 20 million calls were made by PSRs to physicians and pharmacists (Ransom, 2017). But there are many studies where the researchers found the impact is not significant enough (Jamshed et al., 2012; Narendran and Narendranathan, 2013; Biswas and Ferdousy, 2016). It might be because physicians get huge direct marketing communication from pharmaceutical companies every day and therefore, the pharmaceutical companies have failed to gain physicians' interest in a more favorable way. Physicians can be judgmental on receiving calls and other direct communications from PSRs, otherwise pharmaceutical companies need to rethink about applying such direct channels.

CHAPTER 7

Guidelines for Ethical practices

7.1. Overview

This chapter explains the research findings' applicability. Besides that, this chapter shows an effort to understand the elements contributing to physicians' prescription behaviour. A complete approach for measuring the behaviour also emphasizes the importance of moral judgment factor associated with it. The proposed relationships between the constructs were discussed in the previous chapters. This chapter then considers the findings to explain the study's suggestions and consequences by introducing stringent guidelines for pharmaceutical marketers, medical regulatory policymakers and specially physicians for ethical practices.

7.2. Guideline for Pharmaceutical Marketers

For product managers in pharmaceutical companies, the issue is to understand how prescribers will response to the different components of promotional mix that are directed towards them. Medicine prescribers are the customers of pharmaceutical companies and if management can understand their responses better than the promotional war going on in the market, then it will be a potentially significant source of competitive advantage for pharmaceutical companies.

Now that the response has been explored from this study, the product managers must work on reorganizing their communication channels to carry it. Direct marketing channels (direct call, SMS, mobile apps, e-mail and postal mail) are less effective for the physicians. So, the advertising and promotional budgets regarding direct marketing channels can be released. Reducing product promotional budget will eventually decrease the cost of goods sold (COGS) of that product and pricing. Physicians will be prescribing more of the product which is not overly priced. A wide range of consumers (patients) can be targeted when patient centricity is the goal of pharmaceutical business by offering a competitive pricing of medicines in the market.

Pharmaceutical sales representatives (PSRs) get rarely ten minutes time for visiting a physician (Kotler, 2002). As face to face interactions are not possible in emergency situations like happened in Covid-19 era, personal selling will be more difficult and expensive to conduct. Therefore, the pharmaceutical industry should strictly comply with the guidelines as physicians are the direct front liners in any pandemic situations. Pharmaceutical companies should focus on alternative communication channels which are permitted by the regulatory authorities to conduct personal selling, for example, online platform (Google Meet, Microsoft Team, Cisco WebEx) to interactively visit a medical doctor in a timely fashion. If pharmaceutical associations can organize such collective online meeting, then it will save time for the physicians rather than individual meeting. This can be followed beside contingency plan in any pandemic situation as the lessons learnt from Covid-19.

Advertising product brochures and leaflets can be distributed online transforming the print media to online media. The cost of print media can be dissolved resulting release of more allocated budget. Providing gifts to physicians can be scrutinized as sales promotion has been found the most significant factor influencing physicians. Any type of sales promotion (gifts, drug samples, etc.) can be provided upon regulatory permission and physicians' approval. Some physicians are reluctant to receive gifts. So, it is better to offer those who are not reluctant. A drop box of physical gimmick items (pen, writing pad, etc.) addressing physician's name on it can be put in the hospitals, clinics, and other medical centers where physicians usually practice. All these channels are used in the hope of getting more prescription of branded medicines (Kotler, 2002).

7.3. Guideline for Medical Regulatory Bodies

Globally, many developing countries have codes of ethics for pharmaceutical marketing practices. Developed countries like USA and some European countries accomplished regulations on pharmaceutical companies to disclose payment information to physicians. Multinational pharmaceutical companies mostly have their own code of ethics. Malaysia depends primarily on industry self-regulation of promotional practices, but eventually the regulatory bodies under the Ministry of Health (MOH) are liable for enforcing the law. Although strict regulations are in place by the PhAMA (Pharmaceutical Association of Malaysia) Code of Pharmaceutical Marketing Practices for Prescription (Ethical) Products, some recommendations can be made for the regulatory bodies to improve. For instance, medical regulatory bodies should enforce pharmaceutical companies to disclose officially in their online portal about any type of payment (travel, meals, accommodation, registration fees, and honorarium) information received by the healthcare professionals. Pharmaceutical member companies should deploy external audit firms besides self-auditing (internal audit) to investigate any violations of the code of ethics on a regular interval. Formal official-complaints of breaching the code of conduct should be treated by the ethics committee in a minimum period of time. When the pharmaceutical companies breaching the code of conduct again and again, instead of applying penalty, regulators should cancel the licenses for repeat offenders and make the non-compliant pharmaceutical company information publicly available so that healthcare professionals are aware of it. Regulatory bodies should establish mandatory requirements for pharmaceutical sales representatives and healthcare professionals to undertake moral education before practicing.

7.4. Guideline for Healthcare Professionals

Schaefer and Savulescu (2017) from University of Oxford offered a practical guide on moral judgment which has been adapted here based on the results of this study. The guide has been suggested considering physicians' cognitive, self-management, social and motivational abilities to increase for better moral judgment. Physicians' should care about making good, reliable judgments if they care about doing the right thing. This guide will help physicians to facilitate their moral judgment. Oftentimes, physicians' make split-second decisions while prescribing medicines and even in that time they must think procedures to produce good, reliable results. The guidelines for physicians centered two crucial steps as below:

1. Assisting in clear discussion over moral subjects; and
2. Assisting in clear discussion over how one can be most moral when careful discussion over moral subjects is not possible.

Thus, good judgment can regulate moral decision-making in physicians' prescription behaviour. The guideline for physicians can be as follows:

1. Physicians need to have moral consciousness to identify inconsistencies and unethical behaviour governing their interaction with pharmaceutical sales representatives. It is necessary to recognize a moral fault in the beginning of a relationship.
2. Moral ideas are usually complicated, and therefore, physicians should have clear and distinct ideas on moral issues. Even when they write the prescription,

doubts may arise. If physicians are morally judgmental then moral judgment must settle down these doubts and produce fair prescriptions.

3. Physicians need to prioritize the relative importance of competing moral issues and considerations. For example, while prescribing, what is more important for a physician, reputation of the drug manufacturer or the drug quality? Physicians should manage setting priorities as to such moral questions to consider in the first place.
4. Physicians need to have self-control on their intentional actions and actual judgments. For example, physicians might recognize the moral imperative to prescribe less expensive and/or more effective drugs, yet, prescribing the ones which are more expensive and/or less effective. Such kind of weakness in prescription behaviour can be reduced by having self-control to consciously-held moral judgments.
5. Biasness is very common in prescription behaviour which manipulates physicians' moral way of thinking. For example, prescribing the highly promoted medicine irrespective of quality and/or sufficient clinical evidences. Therefore, physicians need to be aware for avoiding such unethical behaviour.
6. Physicians can use more systematic approach (for example, decision procedures) to deal with certain problems like bias. Moral judgment requires further engagement with such decision procedures - awareness of the interest, and willingness to avoid such interest.
7. Physicians should expose pharmaceutical sales representatives to factors that have been overlooked before. This is called dialectical skills which can be accomplished into two ways: reception and communication. Reception means the capacity to fairly and accurately appreciate what PSRs are offering in the promotions and communication corresponds to fairly and accurately communicating the promotional offerings to other physicians.
8. Physicians should have the ability to recognize and evaluate the state of mind of others. This will allow them to engage in moral deliberation considering the personal interest of others in various situations. This will help to avoid self-serving biases towards ensuring responsible prescription behaviour.
9. Moral judgment not always depends on the good fortune of interaction with specific idealized persons; some consequences may seem far away or uncertain. For example, the efficacy of a newly launched medicine promoted by the PSRs. Therefore, the assessment of the fairly imagined arguments (possible side-effects) can take the form of an arrangement for prescribing such medicines for the physicians to be dealt with, one way or the other.

10. Physicians should demonstrate openness or prompt moral reflection to revise their prescription behaviour. It is useless if, upon finding a mistake, a physician is unwilling to correct the error. Therefore, openness to revision may lead to willingness to change one's judgments and ultimately, behaviour.
11. Any improvement is a continuous process. In prescription behaviour, physicians can also seek support from new sources of knowledge, online literatures, and willingness to deliberate their duties more effectively. Expert comments from key opinion leaders in medical profession are important to gain improvement.
12. Finally, if physicians really care about serving their patients then they must have demonstrated a certain degree of moral courage. For example, serving their duties in a pandemic situation like Covid-19 where their own lives are at stake. It is sometimes hard to pursue the right course of action. Therefore, physicians with strong moral courage will stick to their path irrespective of any situation.

7.5. Contribution

There is a lack of theoretical contribution in prescription behaviour studies challenged by the aggressive promotional activity (stimulus) by pharmaceutical companies towards physician's moral decision which is inherent to appropriate prescription behaviour (response). In 1927, Ivan Pavlov (1849-1936) directed perhaps one of the most renowned psychological experiments by arranging a stimulus to have a predictive relationship with reinforce which results in a change in responding to the stimulus (Hogarth, 2013; McLeod, 2014). This becomes known as Stimulus-Response Theory of Behavior. Another great scholar, Dr. Philip Kotler introduced buyer behaviour model and named after Pavlovian stimulus response theory. Based on the model developed by Kotler (2003), while using the deontological theory of ethics; this study carries a major contribution by fulfilling the research gaps in the area of prescription behaviour, and in the area of morality, which is cross-disciplinary in nature. Prescription behaviour and ethical dilemma are the two most found output effects between drug prescribers and pharmaceutical companies (Latten et al., 2018).

This book offers a comprehensive understanding of the factors that influence physicians' prescription decision making, and how these factors, namely: advertising, sales promotion, personal selling, public relations, direct marketing and moral judgment are interrelated in the context of prescription behaviour. It integrates moral behaviour (Reynolds and Ceranic, 2007) with buyer behaviour (Kotler, 2003) by incorporating moral judgment into the study of physicians' prescription behaviour. This research discusses the interaction effects of moral judgment between pharmaceutical promotional mix factors and physicians' prescription behaviour which are also primitive to explain physicians' prescription behaviour.

Therefore, in view of the theoretical and practical contribution of this study, academicians may scrutinize prescription behaviour from a new perception and work in association with other industry partners to direct future research into physicians' moral behaviour in prescribing medicines. This study makes several contributions to the management of pharmaceutical marketing in terms of promotion directed towards physicians. With intense growth of the pharmaceutical industry, physicians are highly influenced by pharmaceutical promotion and experiencing ethical dilemma. As a result, prescription drugs are becoming less effective, more expensive and sometimes are not really needed by the patients.

This study will help the pharmaceutical business to develop more effective plans to gain competitive advantage for their business by having a guideline for pharmaceutical marketers, as an input to the more efficient allocation of their promotional budgets. The guideline is discussed in the recommendation section. This study could potentially increase physicians' awareness about their moral behaviour while prescribing, thus eradicating ethical dilemma and considering appropriate prescription behaviour. They will gain concern governing their interactions with the pharmaceutical sales representatives. As a result, healthcare service quality will increase, and physicians will gain trust from patients. Physicians' moral behaviour will push pharmaceutical companies to maintain ethical relationships and it will increase their reputation resulting in physicians' satisfaction and loyalty. Medical regulatory policymakers can obtain information on field level challenges in the interaction between physicians and pharmaceutical sales representatives to control unethical practices. Physicians' prescription behaviour factors are country-specific. This study specially contributes to the pharmacy research priorities given by the Ministry of Health in August 2018 where "Treatment Decision Making" has been prioritized (MOH, 2018).

7.6. Conclusion

The aim of this research was to compile a summary of the literature on the impact of pharmaceutical promotion on medical professionals in the healthcare industry. The issue of ethical predisposition has come in the process. Therefore, the need of theoretical justification with solid background of theories and frameworks both in consumer behaviour and ethics has been researched. After extensive literature review, the researcher came up with a single problem stated that, "physicians who are highly influenced by direct-to-physician promotion can be prone to prescribe medicines which may be less effective, more expensive or that are not really needed by the patients". The objective was not to judge medicine's quality, rather finding to what extent direct-to-physician promotion influences physicians' medicine prescribing decision. The ethical predisposition has been added to extend the research theory for better insights.

The researcher contributed in developing new knowledge which can enrich the academics in prescription behaviour studies and the current practice in promotional spending of pharmaceutical companies. The healthcare industry has a wide range of businesses, sub-industries, and organizations engaged in healthcare-related goods and services. The six key contributors to this field are pharmaceuticals, biotechnology, supplies, manufacturing, hospitals, and regulated health care (Ledesma et al., 2014). Since the last decade, regulated health care has restructured itself in order to thrive in an intolerant environment caused by sector maturation and intensified consumer competitiveness (Kavitha, 2012). Given that the pharmaceutical industry spends the bulk of its advertisement and promotional (A&P) budget on doctors, and the controversy revolves around the effects of such outreach, a crucial concern has emerged about how to resolve this issue. The purpose of this study was to suggest in the field of pharmaceutical promotion and its positive influence on physicians' prescribing actions. As a result of the essential factors that affect physicians' prescribing actions, pharmaceutical firms will need to restructure their existing marketing campaigns and advertising budgets.

The focus of this study was on physicians' drug selection decisions, in light of previous research results that revealed a two-sided relationship between pharmaceutical promotion and physician response. The debate centers on whether medicinal promotion aimed at physicians and moral judgment have any effect on physicians' prescribing conduct. Physicians' moral judgment can have a huge impact on their drug conduct, which can lead to healthier medication prescribing for the benefit of patients. As a result, physicians must be educated in ethical decision-making principles covering their dealings with pharmaceutical sales representatives, such as those developed by the Royal Australian College of Physicians (Othman et al., 2015). To achieve substantial change in the healthcare industry, it is crucial that doctors, pharmaceutical firms, and medical regulatory policymakers understand the challenges and take the recommendations made in this book.

REFERENCES

Abratt, R., & Lanteigne, J. (2000). Factors influencing general practitioners in the prescription of homeopathic medicines. *South African Journal of Business Management*, Vol. 31 No. 3, pp.91-97.

ACT 290. Medicines (Advertisement and Sale) Act 1956 (Revised – 1983). Retrieved from: http://www.pharmacy.gov.my/v2/sites/default/files/document-upload/medicine-advertisement-sale-act-1956-act-290.pdf

ACT 50. Medical Act 1971 as at 1 May 2015. Retrieved from: https://www.mma.org.my/images/pdfs/Link-LawOfMsiaAct/medical-act-1971.pdf

ACT 586. Private Healthcare Facilities and Services Act 1998 as at 1 December 2015. Retrieved from: https://www.mma.org.my/images/pdfs/Link-LawOfMsiaAct/private-healthcare-facilities-and-services-act-1998.pdf

Ahmed, R. R., Streimikiene, D., Abrhám, J., Streimikis, J., & Vveinhardt, J. (2020). Social and Behavioral Theories and Physician's Prescription Behavior. *Sustainability*, Vol. 12 No. 3379, pp. 1-25.

Ahmed, R. R., Vveinhardt, J., & Streimikiene, D. (2018). The direct and indirect impact of Pharmaceutical industry in Economic expansion and Job creation: Evidence from Bootstrapping and Normal theory methods. *The AMFITEATRU ECONOMIC journal*, Vol. 20 No. 48, pp. 454-469.

Ahmed, R. R., Vveinhardt, J., Streimikiene, D., & Awais, M. (2016). Mediating and marketing factors influence the prescription behavior of physicians: An empirical investigation. *Amfiteatru economic*, 18(41), 153-167.

Ajzen, I. (1988). *Attitudes, personality, and behavior*. Chicago: Dorsey Press.

Ajzen, I. (1991). The theory of planned behavior. *Organizational behavior and human decision processes*, 50(2), 179-211.

Ajzen, I., & Fishbein, M. (1975). *Belief, attitude, intention and behavior: An introduction to theory and research.* Addison-Wesley, Reading, MA.

Ajzen, I., & Fishbein, M. (1980). *Understanding attitude and predicting social behavior.* Englewood Cliffs, NJ: Prentice Hall.

Akçura, M. T., & Özdemir, Z. D. (2014). Drug prescription behavior and decision support systems. *Decision support systems*, 57(January 2014), 395-405.

Alam, K., Shah, A., Ojha, P., Palaien, S., & Shankar, P. (2009). Evalaution of drug promotional materials in a hospital setting in Nepal. *Southern med review*, 2(1), 2–6.

Albarq, A. N., & Suleiman, A. K. (2021). Pharmaceutical marketing strategies' influence on physician's prescription behavior. *Archives of Pharmacy Practice*, 12(1),7-12.

Al-dmour, H. H., Al-zu, Z. M. F., & Fahmawi, A. G. (2013). The Inference of the characteristics of pharmaceutical drug advertising upon the level of physicians' acceptance of drugs in Jordan. *International journal of business and management*, 8(9), 63–87.

Al-Hamdi, A. Y., Hassali, M. A. A., & Ibrahim, M. I. M. (2012). Impact of pharmaceutical promotion on healthcare professional's practices and behaviour: Views from general practitioners, medicine dispensers and medical representatives in Yemen. *Journal of Medical Marketing*, Vo. 12 No. 4, pp. 240 246.

Alowi, M., & Kani, Y. (2018). Impact of Pharmaceutical Companies' Promotional Tools on Physicians' Prescription Patterns: A Systematic Review. *Journal of Applied Pharmacy*, Vol. 10 No. 3, pp. 1-10.

Alowi, M., & Kani, Y.A. (2019). Promotion of prescription drugs and its impact on physician's choice behavior. *Journal of pharmaceutical care & health systems*, 6(January 2019), 1-7.

Alves, T. L., Lexchin, J., & Mintzes, B. (2019). Medicines Information and the Regulation of the Promotion of Pharmaceuticals. *Science and Engineering Ethics*, Vol. 25 No. 4, pp. 1167-1192.

Ambler, T. (2000). Marketing metrics. *Business strategy review*, 11(2), 59 - 66.

Andaleeb, S. S., & Tallman, R. F. (1996). Relationships of physicians with pharmaceutical sales representatives and pharmaceutical companies: An exploratory study. *Health marketing quarterly*, 13(4), 79-89.

Anderson, R. (2014). *Pharmaceutical industry gets high on fat profits*. BBC News, 6th November 2014.

Archer, J. C., & McAvoy, P. (2011). Factors that might undermine the validity of patient and multi-source feedback. *Medical education*, *45*(9), 886–893.

Arens, W. F., Weigold, M. F., & Arens, C. (2011). *Contemporary advertising and integrated marketing communications*. (13th ed.). New York: McGraw Hill.

Bagwell, K. (2007). *The economic analysis of advertising*. Handbook of industrial organization, 3, 1701-1844.

Bakthavathsalam, G. (2006). Generic drugs: Cost effective alternate to branded drugs. *Health administrator*, 19(1), 16-19.

Baron, M. W., Pettit, P., & Slote, M. (1997). *Three methods in ethics*. Malden: Blackwell Publishers Inc.

Bazaza, O. (2020). Effect of Pull and Push Marketing Strategies in the Pharmaceutical Field. *International Journal of Business Marketing and Management,* 5(2), 89-99.

Bednarik, J. (2006). Does brand differentiate pharmaceuticals?. *Neuro endocrinology letters*, 26(6), 635-52.

Belch, G. E., & Belch, M. A. (2007). *Advertising and promotion: An integrated marketing communications perspective*. New York: McGraw-Hill.

Bennet, P. D. (2006). *The AMA dictionary of marketing terms*. 2nd ed, New York, McGraw-Hill.

Bere, S. R. D., Bryce, M., Archer, J., Lynn, N., Nunn, S., & Roberts, M. (2014). *Understanding the rise in fitness to practice complaints from members of the public*. Plymouth University Peninsula Schools of Medicine. January 2014.

Berndt, E. R., Bui, L. T., Lucking-Reiley, D. H., & Urban, G. L. (1996), *The roles of marketing, product quality, and price competition in the growth and composition of the US antiulcer drug industry*. in Bresnahan, T.F. and Gordon, R.J. (Eds), The Economics of New Goods, National Bureau of Economic Research, The University of Chicago Press, Chicago, IL, 277-328.

Bettinghaus, E. P. (1980). *Persuasive communication*. New York: Holt, Rinehart and Winston. ISBN: 978-0030553523.

Bhatt, P. (2018). Study on Influence of Medical Representative in Conversation of Doctor's Prescription in India. *Global Journal of Management and Business Research*, Vol. 18 No. 3, Version 1.0.

Biswas, K., & Ferdousy, U. K. (2016). Influence of Pharmaceutical Marketing on Prescription Behavior of Physicians: A Cross-sectional Study in Bangladesh. *Journal of Accounting and Marketing*, Vol. 5 No. 2, 1000160.

Bloomfield, H., Nelson, D., Van Ryn, M., Neil, B., Koets, N., Basile, J., Samaha, F., Kaul, R., Mehta, J., & Bouland, D. (2005). A trial of education, prompts, and opinion leaders to improve prescription of lipid modifying therapy by primary care physicians for patients with ischemic heart disease. *Quality and safety in healthcare*, 14(4), 258-263.

Boltri, J. M., Gordon, E. R., & Vogel, R. L. (2002). Effect of antihypertensive samples on physician prescribing patterns. *Family medicine*, *34*(10), 729–731.

Bradley, S. P., & James, W. (2004). The Pharmaceutical Industry: Challenges in the New Century. *Harvard Business School,* Case No. 703-489.

Brassington, F., & Pettitt, S. (2000). *Principles of marketing*. 2nd Edition, Harlow Pearson Education Limited.

Brax, H., Fadlallah, R., Al-Khaled, L., Kahale, L. A., Nas, H., El-Jardali, F., & Akl, E. A. (2017). Association between physicians' interaction with pharmaceutical companies and their clinical practices: A systematic review and meta-analysis. *PloS one*, Vol. 12 No. 4, e0175493.

Brett, A. S., Burr, W., & Moloo, J. (2003). Are gifts from pharmaceutical companies ethically problematic? A survey of physicians. *Archives of internal medicine*, *163*(18), 2213–2218.

Brigham, A. F., & Linssen, S. (2010). *Your brand reputational value is irreplaceable: Protect it!*. Forbes (February 1, 2010).

Buckley, J. (2006). Pharmaceutical marketing - Time for change. *Electronic journal of business ethics and organization studies*, 9(2), 4-11.

Buusman, A., Andersen, M., Merrild, C., & Elverdam, B. (2007). Factors influencing GPs' choice between drugs in a therapeutic drug group: A qualitative study. *Scandinavian journal of primary health care*, 25(4), 208-213. doi: 10.1080/02813430701652036.

Campbell, E. G., Gruen, R. L., Mountford, J., Miller, L. G., Cleary, P. D., & Blumenthal, D. (2007). A national survey of physician-industry relationships. *The New England journal of medicine*, *356*(17), 1742–1750.

Campo, K., De Staebel, O., Gijsbrechts, E., & Van Waterschoot, W. (2005), Physicians' decision process for drug prescription and the impact of pharmaceutical marketing mix instruments. *Health marketing quarterly*, 22(4), 73-107.

Carey, C., Lieber, E. M. J., & Miller, S. (2015). *Drug firms' payments and physicians' prescribing behavior in Medicare Part D.* NBER Working Papers 26751, National Bureau of Economic Research, Inc.

Caris-Verhallen, W. M., Kerkstra, A., & Bensing, J. M. (1997). The role of communication in nursing care for elderly people: a review of the literature. *Journal of advanced nursing*, 25(5), 915–933.

Carter, F., & Chitturi, R. (2009). Segmentation Based on Physician Behavior: Implications for Sales Forecasting and Marketing-Mix Strategy. *The Journal of Personal Selling and Sales Management,* 29(1), 81-95.

Caudill, T. S., Johnson, M. S., Rich, E. C., & McKinney, W. P. (1996). Physicians, pharmaceutical sales representatives, and the cost of prescribing. *Archives of family medicine*, 5(4), 201-206.

Cegedim (2013). *U.S. Pharmaceutical Company Promotion Spending*. Cegedim Strategic Data 2012. Retrieved from: http://www.skainfo.com/health_care_market_reports/2012_promotional_spending.pdf

Chamberlin, E. (1933). T*he theory of monopolistic competition*. Cambridge, MA: Harvard University Press.

Chew, L. D., O'Young, T. S., Hazlet, T. K., Bradley, K. A., Maynard, C., & Lessler, D. S. (2000). A physician survey of the effect of drug sample availability on physicians' behavior. *Journal of general internal medicine*, *15*(7), 478–483.

Chimonas, S., Brennan, T. A., & Rothman, D. J. (2007). Physicians and drug representatives: Exploring the dynamics of the relationship. *Society of general internal medicine*, 22(2), 184–190.

Chintagunta, P. K., Goettler, R. L., & Kim, M. (2012). New drug diffusion when forward-looking physicians learn from patient feedback and detailing. *Journal of Marketing Research*, 49(6), 807–821.

Chren, M. M., & Landefeld, C. S. (1994). Physicians' behavior and their interactions with drug companies. A controlled study of physicians who requested additions to a hospital drug formulary. *JAMA*, *271*(9), 684–689.

Cialdini, R. B. (1993). *Influence: Science and practice*. 3rd ed., Harper Collins College Publishers: New York, USA.

Clark, M. M., Gong, M., Schork, M., Evans, D., Roloff, D., Hurwitz, M., Maiman, L., & Mellins, R. (1998). Impact of education for physicians on patient outcomes. *American academy of pediatrics*, 101(5), 831–836.

Clow, K., & Baack, D. (2010). *Integrated advertising, promotion, and marketing communications*. Prentice Hall, 27 Dec.

Conner, M., & Armitage, C. J. (1998). Extending the theory of planned behavior: a review and avenues for further research. J*ournal of applied social psychology*, 28(15), 1429–1464.

Couturier, C., Zaleski, I., Jolly, D., & Durieux, P. (2000). Effects of financial incentives on medical practice: Results from a systematic review of the literature and methodological issues. I*nternational journal of quality health care*, 12(2), 133–142.

Crisp, R., & Slote, M. (1997). *Virtue ethics*. Oxford Readings in: Philosophy. Oxford University Press.

Danchev, N., & Nikolova, I. (2007), Generics – present and future. E*ditorial of pharmaceutical biotechnology*, 21(1), 94-99.

Datta, A., & Dave, D. M. (2013). Effects of Physician-Directed Pharmaceutical Promotion On Prescription Behaviors: Longitudinal Evidence. *National Bureau Of Economic Research*, Cambridge, MA 02138.

Dave, D. M. (2013). *Effects of pharmaceutical promotion: A review and assessment.* NBER Working Papers 18830, National Bureau of Economic Research, Inc.

Davis, F. D. (1989). Perceived utility, perceived ease of use, and user acceptance of information technology. *MIS quarterly*, 13(3), 319-340.

De Ferrari, A., Gentille, C., Davalos, L., Huayanay, L., & Malaga, G. (2014). Attitudes and relationship between physicians and the pharmaceutical industry in a public general hospital in Lima, Peru. *PloS one*, *9*(6), e100114. https://doi.org/10.1371/journal.pone.0100114

De Lorme, D. E., Huh, J., Reid, L., & An, S. (2010). The state of public research on over-the-counter drug advertising. I*nternational journal of pharmaceutical and healthcare marketing*. 4(3). 208-231.

Denig, P., Haaijer-Ruskamp, F. M., & Zijsling, D. H. (1988). How physicians choose drug?. *Social science & medicine*, 27(12), 1381-1386.

Diehl, S., Mueller, B., & Terlutter, R. (2008). Consumer responses towards non-prescription and prescription drug advertising in the US and Germany: They don't really like it, but they do believe it. *International Journal of Advertising*, Vol. 27 No. 1, pp. 99-131.

Dixon, D., Takhar, J., Macnab, J., Eadie, J., Lockyer, J., Stenerson, H., François, J., & Bell, M. (2011). Controlling quality in CME/ CPD by measuring and illuminating bias. *The Journal of Continuing Education in the Health Professions*, Vol. 31 No. 2, pp. 109–116.

Dumovic, P., & De Vries, C. (2004), A review of pharmaceutical industry-sponsored medical education: Ten key recommendations for stakeholders. J*ournal of medical marketing*, 4(2), 143-153.

Eccles, M. P., Grimshaw, J. M., Shekelle, P., Schünemann, H. J., & Woolf, S. (2012). Developing clinical practice guidelines: target audiences, identifying topics for guidelines, guideline group composition and functioning and conflicts of interest. *Implementation science: IS*, 7, 60. https://doi.org/10.1186/1748-5908-7-60

Engel, J. F., Blackwell, R. D., & Miniard, P. W. (1986). *Consumer behaviour*, 5th edition. Dryden.

Epstein, A. M., Read, J. L., & Wickoff, R. (1984). Physician beliefs, attitudes and prescribing behavior for anti-inflammatory drugs. A*merican journal of medical sciences*, 77(2), 313-318.

Ferrell, O. C., & Gresham, L. G. (1985). A contingency framework for understanding ethical decision making in marketing. *Journal of marketing,* 49(3), 87-96.

Fickweiler, F., Fickweiler, W., & Urbach, E. (2017). Interactions between physicians and the pharmaceutical industry generally and sales representatives specifically and their association with physicians' attitudes and prescribing habits: A systematic review. *BMJ Open*, 7(9), e016408.

Fiedler, S., & Glöckner, A. (2015). Attention and moral behavior. *Current opinion in psychology*. 6. 139-144. 10.1016/j.copsyc.2015.08.008.

Flynn, L. R., Goldsmith, R. E., & Eastman, J. K. (1994). The king and summers opinion leadership scale: Revision and refinement. *Journal of business research*, 31(1), 55-64.

Frazier, P. A., Tix, A. P., & Barron, K. E. (2004). Testing moderator and mediator effects in counseling psychology research. *Journal of counseling psychology*, 51(2), 157-157.

Gaines-Ross, L. (2008). *Corporate reputation: 12 steps to safeguarding and recovering reputation.* John Wiley & Sons, Hoboken, NJ.

Gallan, A. (2004). Factors that influence physicians' prescribing of pharmaceuticals: A literature review. *Journal of pharmaceutical marketing and management*, 16(4), 3-46.

Ganashree, P., Bhuvana, K., & Sarala, N. (2016). Critical review of drug promotional literature using the World Health Organization guidelines. *Journal of research in pharmacy practice*, 5(3), 162–165.

Garrigan, B., Adlam, A. L. R., & Langdon, P. E. (2018). Moral decision-making and moral development: Toward an integrative framework. *Developmental review*, 49(March 2018), 80–100.

Ghaith, A., Aldmour, H., & Alabbadi, I. (2013). Investigating the Effect of Pharmaceutical Companies' Gifts on Doctors' Prescribing Behavior in Jordan. *European Journal of Social Sciences,* Vol. 36 No 4, pp. 528-536.

Gibson, S. (2014). Regulating direct-to-consumer advertising of prescription drugs in the digital age. *Laws*, 3(3), 410-438.

Godin, G., Bélanger-Gravel, A., Eccles, M., & Grimshaw, J. (2008). Healthcare professionals' intentions and behaviours: a systematic review of studies based on social cognitive theories. *Implementation science: IS*, *3*, 36. https://doi.org/10.1186/1748-5908-3-36

Goncharuk, A. G., & Getman, M. (2014). Benchmarking to improve a strategy and marketing in pharmaceuticals. *Benchmarking: An international journal*, 21(3), 364 – 385.

Granitz, N., & Loewy, D. (2007). Applying ethical theories: Interpreting and responsibility to student plagiarism. *Journal of business ethics*, 72(3), 293-306.

Greene, J. E. (2004). Attention To 'Details': Etiquette and the Pharmaceutical Salesman in Postwar America. *Social Studies of Science*, Vol. 34 No. 2, pp. 271-292.

Groves, R. (2006). Nonresponse rates and nonresponse bias in household surveys. *Public opinion quarterly,* 70(5), 646–675.

Guglielmo S. (2015). Moral judgment as information processing: an integrative review. *Frontiers in psychology*, *6*, 1637. https://doi.org/10.3389/fpsyg.2015.01637

Guldal, D., & Semin, S. (2000). The influences of drug companies' advertising programs on physicians. *International journal of health services*, 30(3), 585–595.

Guo, T., Sriram, S., & Manchanda, P. (2017). Let the sun shine. In: the impact of industry payment disclosure on physician prescription behavior. *Journal of Marketing*, Georgia Tech Scheller College of Business Research Paper No. 17-8.

Gupta, S., Khajuria, K., Khajuria, V., & Kumar, N. (2018). Comparative study of impact of marketing strategies of pharmaceutical houses on prescription practices of doctors rural vs urban. *International Journal of Basic & Clinical Pharmacology,* Vol. 7 No. 5, pp. 1016-1019.

Hailu, A.D., Workneh, B.D. & Kahissay, M.H. (2021). Influence of pharmaceutical marketing mix strategies on physicians' prescribing behaviors in public and private hospitals, Dessie, Ethiopia: A mixed study design. *BMC Public Health,* 21:65, 1-15.

Haines, I. E., & Olver, I. N. (2008). Are self-regulation and declaration of conflict of interest still the benchmark for relationships between physicians and industry?. *The medical journal of Australia*, 189(5), 263-266.

Haque, M. (2020). Aggressive Medicine Promotional Activity of Pharmaceutical Industry All Over the Globe: Who Will Do the Highly Risky Job to Defy the Monstrous Financial Tyrant?. *Bangladesh Journal of Medical Science*, Vol. 19 No. 4, pp. 589-593.

Harrell, G., & Bennet, P. (1974). An evaluation of the expectancy value model of attitude-measurement for physician prescribing behaviour. *Journal of marketing research*, 11(3), 269-78.

Harrison, K. (2014). *Why a good corporate reputation is important to your organization.* Cutting Edge PR (April 5, 2014).

Hassali, M. A., Yuen, K. H., Ibrahim, M. I. M., Wong, J. W., Ng, B. H. and Ho, D. S. S. (2009). Malaysian pharmaceutical industry: Opportunities and challenges. *Journal of Generic Medicines*, Vol. 6 No. 3, pp. 246 – 252.

Helble, M. (2011). The movement of patients across borders: challenges and opportunities for public health. *Bulletin of the World Health Organization*, 89(1), 68–72.

Hemminki E. (1975). Review of literature on the factors affecting drug prescribing. *Social science & medicine*, 9(2), 111–116. https://doi.org/10.1016/0037-7856(75)90103-1

Henderson, J., Miller, G., Pan, Y., & Britt, H. (2008). The effect of advertising in clinical software on general practitioners' prescribing behaviour. *Medical journal of Australia*, 188(1), 15-20.

Hersh, W. R., Crabtree, M. K., Hickam, D. H., Sacherek, L., Friedman, C. P., Tidmarsh, P., Mosbaek, C., & Kraemer, D. (2002). Factors associated with success in searching MEDLINE and applying evidence to answer clinical questions. *Journal of the American Medical Informatics Association: JAMIA*, *9*(3), 283–293. https://doi.org/10.1197/jamia.m0996

Hirschler, B. (2013). *Bribery scandal slashes GlaxoSmithKline's Chinese drug sales*. Thomson Reuters, 23 October.

Hoffman, J. M., Shah, N. D., Vermeulen, L. C, et al. (2009). Projecting future drug expenditures. *American Journal of Health-System Pharmacy*, Vol. 66 No. 3, pp. 237-257.

Hogarth, L. (2013). *Classical (Pavlovian) conditioning*. In: Stolerman I., Price L. (eds) Encyclopedia of Psychopharmacology. Springer, Berlin, Heidelberg.

Hunt, S., & Vitell, S. (1986). A general theory of marketing ethics. *Journal of macromarketing*, 6(1), 5-16.

Ibrahim, I. A. Y., & Bélanger, C. H. (2015). Pharmaceutical Representatives and Prescription Decisions by Physicians in Saudi Arabia. *Journal of Marketing Management*, Vol. 3 No. 2, pp. 69-79.

ICH (2015). *Steering committee meeting report* (29 January 2015) Meeting held on 12 – 13 November 2014, Lisbon, Portugal. Retrieved from: http://www.nifds.go.kr/brd/m_106/down.do?brd_id=board_mfds_448&seq=23991&data_tp=A&file_seq=1

Islam, M. S., & Farah, S. S. (2007). Misleading promotion of drugs in Bangladesh: evidence from drug promotional brochures distributed to general practitioners by the pharmaceutical companies. *Journal of public health*, 29(2), 212–213. https://doi.org/10.1093/pubmed/fdm024

Iyengar, R., Van den Bulte, C., & Valente, T. (2011). Opinion leadership and social contagion in new product diffusion. *Marketing science*, 30(2), 195-211.

Jambulingam, T., Sharma, R., & Ghani, W. (2009). Wealth effects of the pharmaceutical industry-physician interaction compliance guidelines on large pharmaceutical companies. *International journal of pharmaceutical and healthcare marketing*, 3(3), 210 – 235.

James, C., Peabody, J., Solon, O., Quimbo, S., & Hanson, K. (2009). An unhealthy public-private tension: Pharmacy ownership, prescribing, and spending in the Philippines. *Health affairs*, 28(4), 1022-1033.

Jamshed, S. Q., Ibrahim, M. I., Hassali, M. A., Masood, I., Low, B. Y., Shafie, A. A., & Babar, Z. U. (2012). Perception and attitude of general practitioners regarding generic medicines in Karachi, Pakistan: A questionnaire-based study. *Southern med review*, Vol. *5 No.* 1, pp. 22–30.

Janakiraman, R., Dutta, S., Sismeiro, C., & Stern, P. (2008). Physicians' Persistence and Its Implications for Their Response to Promotion of Prescription Drugs. *Management science*, 54(6), 1080-1093.

Joseph, M., Spake, D., & Godwin, D. M. (2008). Aging consumers and drug marketing: senior citizens' views on DTC advertising, the Medicare prescription drug programmers and pharmaceutical retailing. *Journal of medical marketing*, 8(3), 221-228.

Kant, I. (1994). *Ethical philosophy*. 2nd ed., J. W. Ellington, Trans. Indianapolis, IN: Hackett Publishing.

Kant, I. (1998). *Groundwork of the metaphysics of morals*. Edited by Mary Gregor. Cambridge: Cambridge University Press.

Kaptein, M., & Wempe, J. (2002). *Three general theories of ethics and the integrative role of integrity theory*. SSRN Electronic Journal.

Kara-junior, N. (2013). The influence of ethics and good judgment on the controversies of medicine, *Brazilian Journal of Ophthalmology*, 72(6), 359–360.

Katz, D., Caplan, A. L., & Merz, J. F. (2003). All gifts large and small: toward an understanding of the ethics of pharmaceutical industry gift-giving. *The American journal of bioethics,* Vol. 3 No. 3, pp. 39–46.

Kavitha, R. (2012). Health Care Industry in India. *International Journal of Scientific and Research Publications*, Vol. 2 No. 8, pp. 1-4.

Khajuria, A., & Khajuria, V. (2013). Impact of Pharmaceutical marketing communication strategies on prescription practices of physicians. *Research*

Journal of Pharmaceutical, Biological and Chemical Sciences, Vol. 4 No. 3, pp. 882-889.

Khan, N., Naqvi, A., Ahmad, R., Ahmed, F., Mcgarry, K., Fazlani, R., & Ahsan, M. (2016). Perceptions and attitudes of medical sales representatives (MSRs) and prescribers regarding pharmaceutical sales promotion and prescribing practices in Pakistan. *Journal of young pharmacists*, 8(3), 244-250. 10.5530/jyp.2016.3.13.

Khazzaka, M. (2019). Pharmaceutical marketing strategies' influence on physicians' prescribing pattern in Lebanon: Ethics, gifts, and samples. *BMC Health Services Research*, Vol. 19 No. 1, pp. 1-11.

Kim, W. J., & King, K. W. (2009). Product category effects on external search for prescription and nonprescription drugs. *Journal of Advertising*, Vol. 38 No. 1, pp. 5-19.

Kommalage, M., Navanarasie, D., & Basnayake, S. (2016). Scientific research-based evidence used in drug promotion material distributed in Sri Lanka. *Ceylon medical journal*, 61(4), 199.

Kotler, P. (1997). *Marketing Management: Analysis, Planning, Implementation and Control.* (9th ed.), India, Prentice Hall.

Kotler, P. (1999). *Marketing Management.* Prentice Hall of India, New Delhi.

Kotler, P. (2002). *Marketing Management.* 11th ed., Pearson Education International-Prentice Hall marketing, London, UK.

Kotler, P. (2003). *Marketing management.* International Edition: Eleventh, ISBN: 978-0130497154.

Kotler, P. (2004). *Marketing management.* 11th Edition, Pearson Education, pp. 181-183, 187, 189 -193, 196-207.

Kotler, P. (2005). *According to Kotler: The world's foremost authority on marketing answers your Questions.* New York: AMACOM, ISBN: 9780814472958.

Kotler, P., Armstrong, G., Wong, V., & Saunders. (2008). *Principles of marketing.* 5th ed, Essex: Pearson.

Kramer, L., Hirsch, O., Becker, A., & Donner-Banzhoff, N. (2014). Development and validation of a generic questionnaire for the implementation of complex medical interventions. *German medical science: GMS e-journal*, *12*, Doc08. https://doi.org/10.3205/000193

Kumar, R., Hassali, M. A., Kaur, N., & Kader, M. A. (2014). Perceptions of physicians from private medical centers in Malaysia about generic medicine usage: a qualitative study. *Generics and Biosimilars Initiative journal*, Vol. 3 No. 2, pp. 63-70.

Kumar, R., Hassali, M. A., Saleem, F., Alrasheedy, A. A., Kaur, N., Wong, Z. Y., & Kader, M. A. (2015). Knowledge and perceptions of physicians from private medical centres towards generic medicines: a nationwide survey from Malaysia. *Journal of pharmaceutical policy and practice*, Vol. 8 No. 1, pp. 1-13.

Ladeira, W., Dalmoro, M., Maehler, A., & Araujo, C. (2011). Drug prescription practices in Brazil: A structural equation model. *International Journal of Pharmaceutical and Healthcare Marketing*, Vol. 5 No. 4, pp. 262-278.

Lahdesmati, M. (2005). When ethics matters – interpreting the ethical discourse of small nature – based entrepreneurs. *Journal of business ethics*, 61(1), 55-68.

Latten T, Westra D, Angeli F, Paulus A, Struss M, Ruwaard D (2018) Pharmaceutical companies and healthcare providers: Going beyond the gift: An explorative review. *PLoS one*, 13(2), e0191856.

Ledesma, A., McCulloh, C., Wieck, H., & Yang, M. (2014). *Health Care Sector Overview*. Washington State University.

Lee, H., & Yun, Z. (2015). Consumers' perceptions of organic food attributes and cognitive and affective attitudes as determinants of their purchase intentions toward organic food. *Food quality and preference*, 39. 259–267. 10.1016/j.foodqual.2014.06.002.

Lenzer, J. (2016). Two years of sunshine: has openness about payments reduced industry influence in healthcare?. *BMJ,* 354, i4608.

Lexchin, J. (2018). Pharmaceutical company spending on research and development and promotion in Canada, 2013-2016: a cohort analysis. *Journal of Pharmaceutical Policy and Practice*, Vol. 11 No. 5, pp. 1–6.

Lille, W. (1991). *An introduction to ethics*. 3rd ed., Methuen & Co. Ltd.

Lim, C. W., Kirikoshi, T., & Okano, K. (2008). Modeling the effects of physician-directed promotion using genetic algorithm-partial least squares. *International Journal of Pharmaceutical and Healthcare Marketing*, Vol. 2 No. 3, pp. 195-215.

Loudon, D. L., & Bitta, A. J. D. (2002). *Consumer behavior.* 4th ed., Tata McGraw Hill, New Delhi.

Madhavan, S., Amonkar, M. M., Elliott, D., Burke, K., & Gore, P. (1997). The gift relationship between pharmaceutical companies and physicians: An exploratory survey of physicians. *Journal of clinical pharmacy and therapeutics*, 22(3), 207-215.

Mahmoud, A. M. (2016). Consumer trust and physician prescription of branded medicines: An exploratory study. *International journal of pharmaceutical and healthcare marketing*, 10(3), 285-301.

Manchanda, P., & Honka, E. (2005). The effects and role of Direct-to-Physician marketing in the pharmaceutical industry: An integrative review. *Yale journal of health policy, law and ethics*, Vol. 5 No. 2, Article 8.

Matikainen, M., Olkkonen, L., Katajavuori, N., Parvinen, P., & Juppo, A. (2017). Physicians' relationship with the pharmaceutical industry and its reflection in introduction of a new drug. *International journal of pharmaceutical and healthcare marketing*, 11(3), 309-326.

McCarthy, E. J. (1960). *Basic marketing, a managerial approach*. IL: Richard D. Irwin.

McKinney, W. P., Schiedermayer, D. L., Lurie, N., Simpson, D. E., Goodman, J. L., & Rich, E. C. (1990). Attitudes of internal medicine faculty and residents toward professional interaction with pharmaceutical sales representatives. *JAMA*, 264(13), 1693-1697.

McLeod, S. A. (2014). *Classical conditioning*. Retrieved from: www.simplypsychology.org/classical-conditioning.html

Medicines Australia. (2007). *Code of conduct.* Edition 15. Retrieved from: http://www.medicinesaustralia.com.au/pages/page254.asp.

Meo, A., Abbas, M., Sajjad, M., Rizwan, M., bukhari, S., & Hameed, M. (2014). The impact of promotional tools on sales promotion. *Journal of public administration and governance, 4*(2), 202-216.

MIDA (2018). *Malaysian Investment Development Authority: Annual Report.* Retrieved from: https://www.mida.gov.my/home/administrator/system_files/modules/photo/uploads/20200204083911_MIDA_AR2018_Eng_Final.pdf

Mintzes, B., Lexchin, J., Sutherland, J. M., Beaulieu, M. D., Wilkes, M. S., Durrieu, G., et al. (2013). Pharmaceutical sales representatives and patient safety: a comparative prospective study of information quality in Canada, France and the United States. *Journal of general internal medicine*, 28(10), 1368-1375.

Mizik, N., & Jacobson, R. (2004). Are physicians easy marks? Quantifying the effects of detailing and sampling on new prescriptions. *Management science*, 50(12), 1704-1715.

MOH (2017). *Malaysian statistics on medicines (2011 – 2014).* Ministry of Health, Pharmaceutical Services Division.

MOH (2018). *Ministry of Health: Pharmacy Research Priorities in Malaysia (Reviewed August 2018).* Retrieved from: https://www.pharmacy.gov.my/v2/sites/default/files/document-upload/pharmacy-research-priorities-malaysia-2018.pdf

Mohammed, R., & Kheder, S. (2017). The impact of pharmaceutical promotion on rational prescribing and drug use in Sudan. *Sudan Medical Monitor*, Vol. 12 No. 1, pp. 19-23.

Murshid, M. A., & Mohaidin, Z. (2017). Models and theories of prescribing decisions: A review and suggested a new model. *Pharmacy Practice*, Vol. 15 No. 2, 990.

MyCC (2017). *Malaysia Competition Commission: Market Review on Priority Sector under Competition Act 2010 – Pharmaceutical Sector.* Retrieved from: https://www.mycc.gov.my/sites/default/files/pdf/newsroom/Market%20Review%20on%20Pharmaceutical%20Sector.pdf

Narayanan, S., Manchanda, P., & Chintagunta, P. K. (2005). Temporal differences in the role of marketing communication in new products categories. *Journal of marketing research*, 42(August), 278–290.

Narendran, R., & Narendranathan, M. (2013). Influence of pharmaceutical marketing on prescription practices of physicians. *The Journal of the Indian Medical Association*, Vol. 111 No. 1, pp. 47-50.

Negash, M., & Adamu, A. (2017). The Impact of Pharmaceutical Promotion Strategies on Prescribing Behavior of Physicians A Developing Country Experience: Case of Addis Ababa, Ethiopia. *Pacific Business Review International*, Vol. 9 No. 8, pp. 9–18.

Neil, O., & Patrick, M. (1995). *Ethics*. In: John, K.R. (ed), International Encyclopedia of Ethics. London: Fitzroy Dearborn Publishers, pp: 281.

O'Guinn, C. T., Allen, C. T., & Semenik, R. J. (2009). *Advertising & integrated brand promotion*, 5th Ed., SouthWestern Cengage Learning: USA.

O'keefe, D. J. (2002). *Persuasion: theory and research*. Thousand Oaks, CA: SAGE. ISBN: 978-0761925392.

Othman, N., Vitry, A. I., Roughead, E. E. *et al.* (2010). Medicines information provided by pharmaceutical representatives: A comparative study in Australia and Malaysia. *BMC Public Health,* 10, 743 (2010). https://doi.org/10.1186/1471-2458-10-743

Othman, N., Vitry, A. I., Roughead, E. E., Ismail, S. B., & Omar, K. (2015). Doctors' Views on The Quality Of Claims Provided By Pharmaceutical Representatives: A Comparative Study In Malaysia And Australia. *Journal of Taibah University Medical Sciences*, Vol. 10 No. 4, pp. 471-480.

Ouwersloot, H., & Duncan, T. (2008). *Integrated marketing communications*. (European edition). McGraw-Hill, London.

Pearsall, J. (1999). *The concise oxford dictionary*. 10 ed., Oxford University Press, pp: 489-490.

Pellegrino, E. D. (1994). Ethics. *JAMA*, 271, 1668–1670.

Percy, L., & Richard, R-E. (2016). *Strategic advertising management.* 5th Ed, Oxford, England: Oxford University Press.

Perkins, M. B., Jensen, P. S., Jaccard, J., Gollwitzer, P., Oettingen, G., Pappadopulos, E., Hoagwood, K. E. (2007). Applying theory-driven approaches to understanding and modifying clinicians' behavior: What do we know?. *Psychiatric services*, 58(3), 342-348.

Pettifor, J. L., Estay, I., & Paque, S. (2000). Preferred strategies for learning ethics in the practice of a discipline. *Canadian psychology*, 43(4), 260-269.

Petty, R. E., & Cacioppo, J. T. (1986). *The Elaboration Likelihood Model of Persuasion.* In: Communication and Persuasion. Springer Series in Social Psychology. Springer, New York, NY. https://doi.org/10.1007/978-1-4612-4964-1_1

Pezzola, A., & Sweet, C. M. (2016). Global pharmaceutical regulation: the challenge of integration for developing states. *Global Health,* 12, 85.

PhAMA Code of Conduct (2019). *Pharmaceutical Marketing Practices for Prescription (Ethical) Products.* The pharmaceutical association of Malaysia, 21st edition.

Piong, J., & Loong, C. M. (2014). Malaysia Pharmaceutical Industry – Collaboration and Investment Opportunities. *Journal of Pharmaceutical Machinery and Engineering*, Vol. 23 No.1, pp. 1-11.

Planchon, J. M., James, W. L., & Van-Hoof, L. (2009). Believability of informational versus transformational prescription drug advertising: US consumers' views versus Belgian consumers' views. *Review of Business Research*, Vol. 9 No. 4, pp. 183-8.

Ponnet, K., Wouters, E., Van Hal, G., Heirman, W., & Walrave, M. (2014). Determinants of physicians' prescribing behaviour of methylphenidate for cognitive enhancement. *Psychology, health and medicine*, 19(3), 286-295.

Premeaux, S. R. (2004). The current link between management behavior and ethical philosophy. *Journal of business ethics*, 51(May 2004), 269-278.

Prosser, H., Almond, S., & Walley, T. (2003). Influences on GPs' decision to prescribe new drugs – the importance of who says what. *Family practice*, 20(1), 61-68.

Punchibandara, M. M. T. (2017). The impact of promotional strategies of pharmaceutical companies on doctor' s recommendation of branded drugs: An empirical study in Sri Lanka. *Kelaniya journal of management,* (Special Issue), 55-66.

Rahman, M. K., Khan, A. H., & Jalil, A. (2014). Ethical implications of sales promotion in Malaysia. *Islamic perspective*, 2(1), 13–27.

Raisch, D. W. (1990). A model of methods for influencing prescribing: A review of educational methods, theories of human inference and delineation of a model. *Annals of pharmacotherapy*, 24(5), 537-542.

Ransom, A. B. (2017). *Direct-to-Physician Advertising, Depression, and the Advertised Female Patient*. PhD dissertation, University of Tennessee.

Rasekh, H. R., Mehralian, G., & Vatankhah-Mohammadabadi, A. A. (2012). Situation analysis of R &D activities: An empirical study in Iranian pharmaceutical companies. *Iranian journal of Pharmaceutical Research*, Vol. 11 No. 4, pp. 1013–1025.

Rashidian, A., Miles, J., Russell, D., & Russell, I. (2006). Sample size for regression analyses of theory of planned behaviour studies: case of prescribing in general practice. *British journal of health psychology*, 11(Pt 4), 581–593. https://doi.org/10.1348/135910705X66043

Reidenbach, R. E., & Robin, D. P. (1988). Some initial steps toward improving the measurement of ethical evaluations of marketing activities. *Journal of business ethics*, 7(11), 871-879.

Rest, J. R. (1986). *Moral development: Advances in research and theory*. New York: Praeger.

Reyna, V. F., & Rivers, S. E. (2008). Current theories of risk and rational decision making. *Developmental review*, 28(1), 1-11. doi: 10.1016/j.dr.2008.01.002.

Reynolds, S. J., & Ceranic, T. L. (2007). The effects of moral judgment and moral identity on moral behavior: An empirical examination of the moral individual. *The Journal of applied psychology*, 92(6), 1610–1624.

Rivero, O., & Theodore, J. (2014). The importance of public relations in corporate sustainability. *Global journal of management and business research (B)*, 14(4), version 1.

Rockoff, J. D. (2012). *Drug reps soften their sales pitches.* Wall street journal, January 10, 2012.

Rosnah, N., & Abdullah, W. (2002). Medical Regulation in Malaysia: Towards an Effective Regulatory Regime. *Policy, Organization and Society*, 21(1), 96-124.

Salmasi, S., Ming, L. C., & Khan, T. M. (2016). Interaction and medical inducement between pharmaceutical representatives and physicians: A meta-synthesis. *Journal of pharmaceutical policy and practice,* 9, 37 (2016).

Salmasi, S., Ming, L. C., & Khan, T. M. (2016). Interaction and medical inducement between pharmaceutical representatives and physicians: A meta-synthesis. *Journal of pharmaceutical policy and practice,* 9, 37 (2016). https://doi.org/10.1186/s40545-016-0089-z

Sanyal, S. N., Datta, S. K., & Banerjee, A. K. (2017). Factors influencing prescribing decisions among physicians: an empirical study on generic drugs. *International Journal of Pharmaceutical and Healthcare Marketing*, Vol. 11 No. 4, pp. 330-360.

Schaefer, G. O., & Savulescu, J. (2016). Procedural moral enhancement. *Neuroethics,* 12, 73–84. https://doi.org/10.1007/s12152-016-9258-7

Schommer, J. C., & Hansen, R. A. (2005). The study of direct-to-consumer advertising for prescription drugs. *Research in social and administrative pharmacy*, 1(2), 348-368.

Segal, R., & Hepler, D. C. (1982). Prescribers' beliefs and values as predictors of drug choices. *American journal of hospital pharmacy*, 39(11), 1891-1897.

Shamim-ul-Haq, S., Ahmed, R. R., Ahmad, N., Khoso, I., & Parmar, V. (2014). Factors Influencing Prescription Behavior of Physicians. *The Pharma Innovation Journal*, Vol. 3 No. 5, pp. 30-35.

Sharifnia, H. S. A., Mohammadzadeh, M., Arzani, G., Salamzadeh, J., Abolfazli, S. A., Zali, A., & Khoshdel, A. R. (2018). Main factors affecting physicians' prescribing decisions: The Iranian experience. *Iranian journal of pharmaceutical research*, 17(3), 1105-1115.

Sisugoswami, M., Al- Shiibami, A. H., & Nusari, M. S. (2018). Attitude of physician towards gift acceptance from the representatives of pharmaceutical company and its impact on prescription pattern in Malaysia. *International Journal on Recent Trends in Business and Tourism*. 2(2), pp. 33-39.

Skandrani, H., & Sghaier, M. (2016). The dark side of the pharmaceutical industry. *Marketing intelligence & planning*, 34(7), 905-926.

Smetana, J. G. (2013). *Moral development: The social domain theory view. In: P. D. Zelazo (Ed.),* Oxford library of psychology. The Oxford handbook of developmental psychology (Vol. 1): Body and mind *(p. 832–863). Oxford University Press.*

Stafford, R. S., Furberg, C. D., Finkelstein, S. N., Cockburn, I. M., & Alehegn, T. (2004). Impact of clinical trial results on national trends in alpha-blocker prescribing, 1996–2002. *JAMA,* 291, 54–62.

Statista Report (2015). *Revenue of the worldwide pharmaceutical market from 2001 to 2015 (in billion U.S. dollar).* Retrieved from: https://www.statista.com/statistics/263102/pharmaceutical-market-worldwide-revenue-since-2001/

Thomas, L. S., & Valli, A. (2006). Levels of occupational stress in doctors working in a South African public-sector hospital. *South African medical journal forum*, 96 (11), 1162-1168.

Thomson, A. N., Craig, B. J., & Barham, P. M. (1994). Attitudes of general practitioners in New Zealand to pharmaceutical representatives. *The British journal of general practice: the journal of the Royal College of General Practitioners*, 44(382), 220–223.

Trevino, L. K. (1992). Moral reasoning and business ethics: Implications for research, education and management. *Journal of business ethics*, 11(5/6), 445-459.

Turiel, E. (1983). *The development of social knowledge: Morality and convention.* Cambridge: Cambridge University Press.

Uusitalo, L. (2010). *Advertising and consumer behavior.* In: Consumer behaviour (Chapter 28), Publisher: Lund.

Velasquez, M. G. (1992). *Business ethics: Concepts and cases.* New Jersey: Prentice Hall. Third edition: pp.62-63.

Ventola C. L. (2011). Direct-to-Consumer Pharmaceutical Advertising: Therapeutic or Toxic?. *P & T: a peer-reviewed journal for formulary management*, 36(10), 669–684.

Waheed, K. A., Jaleel, M., & Laeequddin, M. (2011). Prescription loyalty behavior of physicians: an empirical study in India. *International Journal of Pharmaceutical and Healthcare Marketing*, Vol. 5 No. 4, pp. 279-298.

Wazana A. (2000). Physicians and the pharmaceutical industry: is a gift ever just a gift?. *JAMA*, *283*(3), 373–380.

Wei, M., & Delbaere, M. (2015). Do consumers perceive their doctors as influenced by pharmaceutical marketing communications? A persuasion knowledge perspective. *International journal of pharmaceutical and healthcare marketing*, 9(4), 330 – 348.

Weiss, J., (2010). Medical marketing in the United States: A prescription for reform. *The George Washington law review*, 79(1), 260-292.

Wendy, D., & Herman, S. (2007). *Healthcare: Pharmaceuticals.* Standard & Poor's Corporation: Industry Surveys, 22 December 2007.

WHO (World Health Organization, 1988) *Ethical criteria for medicinal drug promotion.* Geneva: World Health Organization.

Williams, J. R., & Hensel, P. J. (1991). Changes in physicians' sources of pharmaceutical information: A review and analysis. *Journal of health care marketing*, 11(3), 46–60.

Wilson, D. R. (2005). *The six simple principles of viral marketing.* Retrieved from: http://www.wilsonweb.com/wmt5/viral-principles.htm

Wittich, C. M., Burkle, C. M., & Lanier, W. L. (2014). Medication errors: An overview for clinicians. *Mayo clinic proceedings*. 89(8), 1116-1125.

Wittink, D. R. (2002). *Analysis of ROI for Pharmaceutical Promotions (ARPP).* In: Presentation to the Association of Medical Publications.

Workneh, B. D., Gebrehiwot, M. G., Bayo, T. A., Gidey, M. T., Belay, Y. B., Tesfaye, D. M., et al. (2016). Influence of Medical Representatives on Prescribing Practices in Mekelle, Northern Ethiopia. *PLoS ONE,* Vol. 11 No. 6, e0156795.

Wozniak, L., Hassan, M., & Benner, D. (2012). Changing paradigms in the long-term care market Perspective of the pharmaceutical industry. *International journal of pharmaceutical and healthcare marketing*, 6(3), 267 – 278.

Xing, J. L., & Othman, M. H. (2015). Rational decision-making models might suggest what people ought to do, they are a poor guide to what people actually do. *International Journal of Accounting, Business & Management*, Vol. 1 No. 1, pp. 1-5.

Zahrani, H. (2014). The impact of pharmaceutical promotions on primary health care physicians' prescribing behaviour in KAMC in central region. *International Journal of Medical Science and Public Health*, Vol. 3 No. 3, pp. 358-364.

Zaki, N. M. (2014). Pharmacists' and physicians' perception and exposure to drug promotion: A Saudi study. *Saudi pharmaceutical journal: the official publication of the Saudi Pharmaceutical Society*, *22*(6), 528–536.

Zetterqvist, A. V., Merlo, J., & Mulinari, S. (2015). Complaints, Complainants, and Rulings Regarding Drug Promotion in the United Kingdom and Sweden 2004–2012: A Quantitative and Qualitative Study of Pharmaceutical Industry Self-Regulation. *PLoS med,* 12(2), e1001785.

www.ingramcontent.com/pod-product-compliance
Lightning Source LLC
LaVergne TN
LVHW022309200926
848481LV00004B/1248
9798892488877